Cancer

Special Diet Cookbook

Cancer

Special Diet Cookbook

Over 100 recipes to help overcome eating difficulties and enjoy a healthy diet

Clare Shaw and Maureen Hunter

Thorsons
An Imprint of HarperCollins*Publishers*

Thorsons
An Imprint of GraftonBooks
A Division of HarperCollins*Publishers*
77-85 Fulham Palace Road,
Hammersmith, London W6 8JB

Published by Thorsons 1991
1 3 5 7 9 10 8 6 4 2

Clare Shaw and Maureen Hunter assert
the moral right to be identified
as the authors of this work

A catalogue record for this book
is available from the British Library

ISBN 0 7225 2406 4

Typeset by Harper Phototypesetters Limited,
Northampton, England
Printed in Great Britain by
The Bath Press, Bath, Avon

Contents

Acknowledgements

We are grateful to the following friends and colleagues who helped us devise and test the recipes: our mothers, Barbara and Sue Davis, Virginia Souchon, Jackie Green, Grace and Renée Bevan, Ruth Abraham, Pat Crooks and Robert Williams.

We would also like to acknowledge the hard work and efficiency of David Proudfoot who typed his way through the text and over 100 recipes.

About the Authors

Clare Shaw and Maureen Hunter are qualified dietitians and experts in nutrition. They have special knowledge of the nutritional aspects of cancer care having several years' experience as dietitians, working with cancer patients with eating difficulties, at a leading London cancer hospital.

Foreword

Good nutrition plays an essential role in the treatment of cancer: not only does it assist people to withstand the effects of treatment, it is a crucial component in aiding recovery once the treatment has been completed.

In recent years there has been a much greater emphasis on nutrition and cancer — especially the so-called 'alternative' diets, some of which have claimed to have a curative effect on the disease. This has sometimes caused confusion and dismay for those who did not fully understand the debate. This book clearly explains these diets and goes further in offering sensible advice for people with cancer who are contemplating undertaking them.

An essential aspect of cancer care today is that the patient is informed, that he or she has sufficient information to participate in treatment decisions and manage its side-effects, and this applies as much to diet as to any other aspect of treatment.

This excellent book helps cancer patients achieve this partnership in their care as far as nutrition is concerned and contains a wealth of important information to enable the individual to eat well and enjoyably throughout treatment and beyond.

The information contained within this book, together with the wide range of recipes to meet most nutritional needs, should ensure a continuance of one of life's greatest pleasures — eating! Bon appetit!

Richard J. Wells, FRCN
Head of Rehabilitation Services,
Marie Curie Rehabilitation Unit,
The Royal Marsden Hospital

Introduction

Nutrition is now recognized as being an important factor in the overall treatment of patients with cancer as many patients experience eating difficulties during treatment. Sometimes these are short-term, minor problems; sometimes they last longer and cause problems with maintaining weight and nutritional status. For all cancer patients, though — whether they have problems with eating or not — there is much conflicting and confusing information available as to what sort of food should be eaten. In this book, however, you will find clear guidelines for the patient, their relatives and carers on all aspects of nutrition and cancer.

The first chapter looks at the evidence to date on the links between diet and causation of cancer. This clarifies the confusion that has arisen from some current publications and the press, causing extra anxiety to newly diagnosed patients. The chapter explains how diet is just one of numerous risk factors in cancer development, many of which remain unknown.

The second chapter examines the concepts of healthy eating for those patients who are yet to start treatment, for those whose appetite is not affected during treatment or for those who have completed treatment and are eating normally. The chapter also includes detailed advice for those who are experiencing eating difficulties at any time.

The third discusses various complementary dietary therapies that are popular with some patients. The most used regimes are outlined to enable the reader to make an informed choice as to their suitability in their own circumstances.

Over 100 tasty recipes, suitable for both healthy eating and coping with eating difficulties are given in the recipe section. They have been specially designed to taste good and do you good even when you do not have much of an appetite. Those patients who wish to pursue any aspect of this book further will find the suggested reading and information sources at the end of the book very useful.

The Recipes

The recipes are divided into two sections. The first suggests nutritious recipes suitable for those people with eating difficulties, each recipe stating for which eating difficulty it is most suitable. Some of the dessert recipes contain raw eggs, so if you have been informed that you have a low white blood count or you are particularly unwell, do not eat these dishes.

The second section concentrates on recipes for healthy eating with indications in each one as to what particular aspect of healthy eating it addresses. If you are not eating well, however, go ahead and try any of the recipes in the book that take your fancy!

All the recipes give imperial, metric and American measures. To measure an American cupful, fill a measuring jug to the 8 fl oz mark or use the measures made for this purpose — using a mug or coffee cup will not yield satisfactory results. The microwave instructions are for 650W models so adjust the times as necessary if your microwave is more or less powerful. Recipes for dishes that can be frozen have been indicated as such. You will find that most of the recipes are also suitable for the rest of the family.

Spoon measurements used in the recipes are abbreviated as follows:
dsp — dessertspoon
tbs — tablespoon
tsp — teaspoon

Part 1

Diet and Cancer

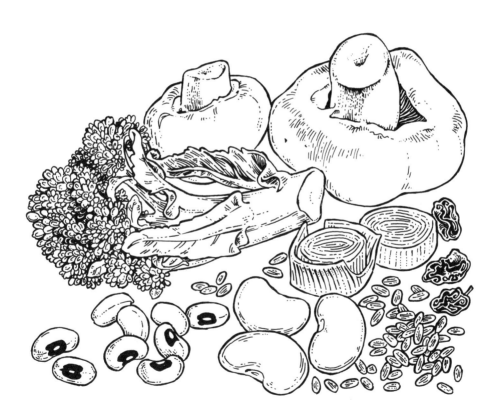

Chapter 1

Links between Diet and Cancer

For many years there has been much interest in and research into what causes cancer. The links between diet and the aetiology, or causation, of cancer are at present not well established, but there follows a brief summary of the chief findings so far. Before we do this, however, let us look at the different ways research into this subject has been carried out and the difficulties investigators have faced in the search for answers. It is known that the rates of various types of cancer are not uniform around the world (in the Western world, for example, we have high rates of breast, large bowel, lung and prostate cancer compared to developing countries). Epidemiological studies have compared rates of cancer incidence in various countries and when these figures were correlated with dietary habits, some possible links between what we eat and cancer risk became evident.

More evidence is provided by animal and clinical studies. The latter are particularly difficult to undertake, however, as it is thought that the role diet plays evolves over many years —

perhaps 20, 30 or more in the case of breast or colon cancer. Also, it is difficult to measure past food intake accurately, especially as many people forget even what they ate the previous day.

It should perhaps also be remembered that cancer affects many different parts of the body. Diet may influence the development of cancer due to food actually coming into contact with organs such as the mouth, oesophagus, stomach and bowel or in other ways that are at present still not known about in sufficient detail, such as hormones, and narrowing down the options is an extremely difficult task. Now to the findings.

Fat

Breast cancer is the most prevalent cancer among women in Britain and, in other Western countries, such as North America where breast cancer rates are high, the total consumption of fat tends also to be high and this has led to investigations into whether there is possibly a link between the two. The Japanese who traditionally eat a diet that is low in fat and meat also have a low incidence of breast cancer. The Japanese diet has gradually changed since the 1950s with an increase in the consumption of fat and it has been observed that the rate of breast cancer in Japan has also risen. Further, it has been found that any influence diet may have on the individual is most likely to occur early in life. Japanese women who emigrated to the United States have an increasing incidence of breast cancer, with higher levels being found in the second generation who had eaten a more Western diet for their entire life.

Epidemiological observations have been supported by animal experiments, some of which date back to the 1930s. However, such evidence can only provide an *indication* of the role of fat. Case-control studies and prospective studies are the best way positively to confirm or refute a link, but, to date, these types of studies have not supported the ideas as much as many researchers had hoped. In addition, attempts to identify which particular types of fat may be important or how a high-fat diet may act have also been unsuccessful as yet. Initial ideas were put forward that diet may raise serum oestrogens, the female sex hormone, as this can, in some cases, stimulate the growth of breast tumours, but, again, clinical studies have not confirmed this. Perhaps more answers will be provided by current work. This research changes the diet of the women in the studies in the hope that they will then be able to determine whether this influences their chances of developing breast cancer.

Bowel cancer and prostate cancer are also prevalent in countries where a relatively high-fat diet is eaten, but, as is the case with breast cancer, human studies have not yet provided conclusive evidence for this kind of diet being a risk factor.

Fibre

Fibre in the diet has enjoyed much publicity in recent years, particularly as eating more of it may lower the risk of various diseases or conditions, especially bowel conditions. Since its initial popularity there has been much debate about the question 'What is fibre?' The latest methods of analysis measure fibres and starch that escape digestion in the small intestine. These substances then pass into the large bowel and, it has been found, act to decrease the length of time the contents of the gut are in contact with the bowel and possibly bind carcinogens or cancer-producing agents.

Dr Denis Burkitt has suggested that fibre in the diet may protect against bowel cancer. His basis for this idea is that rural Africans eat a diet that is bulkier (although recent analysis has shown that it is not necessarily higher in fibre) and Africans have a lower incidence of colon cancer and other digestive disorders. Their diet is also low in fat and meat and these additional factors may be important, as we have seen.

Protein

It is difficult to determine whether high protein intake is linked with various types of cancer. The reasons for this are as follows:

- meat is often used as an indicator of protein consumption and foods containing meat and meat products may also be high in fat
- there are substances present in some meat products that have been implicated as carcinogens
- some cooking methods, particularly those that char or burn foods, such as barbecuing or frying, produce a group of substances known as heterocyclic amines and, while animal studies indicate that these are carcinogenic, it is still not possible to say whether these are detrimental to human beings
- various studies have been unable to show whether or not protein or meat consumption have specific roles in the development of tumours.

Vegetarians do appear to have a reduced risk of developing bowel cancer, but this may be due to additional dietary factors other than avoiding meat.

Alcohol

The strongest association between diet and cancer is between alcoholic drinks and cancer of the head and neck, oesophagus and liver. As early as 1837 it was noted that both smoking and drinking alcohol increased the risk of developing cancer of the tongue. Also, oesophageal cancer was observed to be prevalent among drinkers of pai-san, a strong alcoholic drink, in China, and of home-made apple brandy in Normandy. Finnish alcoholics were found to have a higher rate of cancer of the pharynx compared to the rest of the population. Further, smoking, in addition to being a causative factor in lung cancer, is also a risk factor in oral cancer. Although its effect is independent of alcohol, when taken together, the effects are multiplied.

Some studies have linked large bowel cancer with beer drinking, although findings have not been consistent. As the link does not appear to be with any other alcoholic drinks, it is suggested that other components in beer apart from alcohol may be responsible.

Obesity

Obesity may be a risk factor for breast cancer in post-menopausal women and large bowel cancer in men. However, not all studies have supported these assertions.

Vitamins

There is much interest in the relationship between vitamins and cancer, particularly as they might actually act to protect the body.

Vitamin A and β-Carotene (Beta carotene)

It has been suggested that vitamin A and β-carotene protect individuals from lung cancer. Consumption of the main sources of the vitamins — liver, carrots and green leafy vegetables — was lower in lung cancer patients than in the control groups and the levels of retinol (a source of vitamin A) and β-carotene in the blood were also lower in patients suffering from lung cancer. It is thought, however, that these results may be a consequence of the disease itself rather than a causative factor.

Vitamin A can be found in food as fat-soluble retinol present in liver, fish oils, such as halibut-liver or cod-liver oil, milk, butter and eggs. Alternatively, vitamin A can be made by the body from carotene, principally found as β-carotene, in green leafy vegetables and in some yellow and red fruits or vegetables, for example, apricots, peaches, carrots and sweet potatoes. It is the β-carotene that appears to play a protective role in oesophageal cancer. For example, low intakes of green and yellow vegetables have been linked with high rates of oesophageal cancer in China and Iran. Exactly how β-carotene may protect the body, though, is still unclear. It has been suggested that it may be due to the role of vitamin A in controlling cell division or, perhaps more likely, by acting as an antioxidant. An antioxidant protects fats in the cell membrane from attack, or oxidation, by oxygen molecules. Such oxidation can damage the cell membrane and cause degenerative changes in the cell. A number of studies are now investigating if β-carotene can reduce the incidence of some cancers when given as a dietary supplement. Retinol, however, unlike β-carotene, is toxic if recommended daily allowances are exceeded.

Vitamin C (ascorbic acid)

Epidemiological studies assessing the amount of vitamin C in people's diet have indicated that there may be a link between a low intake of foods high in ascorbic acid content and an increased incidence of oesophageal or stomach cancers and laryngeal cancer. Low levels of ascorbic acid in the blood detected in some patients, though, may simply be due to them eating less food and therefore consuming less vitamin C as a result of their disease.

Vitamin C is known to have a number of important functions within the body. Of particular interest is its ability to act as an antioxidant and inhibit the formation of N-nitroso compounds in laboratory experiments, as these substances can form from nitrates in food and are known to cause cancer in animals and it is likely that the same inhibition occurs in the human stomach. This antioxidant property may protect the cells' DNA, which is required for normal cell replication (DNA, or deoxyribonucleic acid, is a component of cells, essential for cell division).

Vitamin E (α-tocopherol/alpha-tocopherol)

Vitamin E, or α-tocopherol, is a fat-soluble vitamin present in vegetable oils, cereals and eggs. A deficiency in human beings is most unlikely although low levels of α-tocopherol in the blood have been linked with an increased risk in some cancers, such as those of the larynx, oesophagus and stomach.

In epidemiological studies, the intake of vitamins is assessed from the average consumption of fruit and vegetables. There are, however, other compounds present in such foods that may have an influence in cancer development, as we have seen. Others may include flavonoids, tannins, isothiocyanates, found in the cabbage family, phenols and indoles. Some or all of these substances may take part in chemical reactions to enhance the protective effect of vitamins and minerals. If it does appear that fruit and vegetables are protective because of these and other additional compounds then taking vitamin supplements alone would not necessarily help reduce the risk of cancer.

Minerals

Accurate measurements of the intake of minerals in the diet, like vitamins, presents many problems. Minerals, especially trace elements, are present in a wide variety of foods, the concentrations of which can vary greatly depending on where fruits and vegetables are grown. Most of the evidence linking minerals and cancer has originated from animal experimentation.

Selenium

Selenium is a trace element found particularly in cereals, meat and fish. It has been suggested that this mineral can have a protective effect against breast, lung, bowel, prostate, ovarian and bladder cancer, although there is much controversy about the evidence, not all of which is in agreement.

Animal experiments tend to support the idea that selenium may have a protective action.

Studies into how this might work have centred on the antioxidant properties of selenium. It is a necessary component of the enzyme glutathione peroxidase, which helps prevent oxidation of cell lipids or fats, but further investigation has failed to show that larger amounts of selenium present in the diet can activate this enzyme, so investigations continue to search for other possible mechanisms.

Experiments involving dietary supplementation with selenium in humans cannot be carried out due to the toxic nature of this element when taken in excess.

Other minerals

Links between other minerals and the development of cancer are even more tenuous than for selenium intake. Suggestions have been made that some minerals may have a protective effect, including calcium, magnesium, zinc, iron, copper, iodine and molybdenum, but much more research is required before such links can be either confirmed or denied.

Nitrates and Nitrites

As mentioned earlier, it has been found that vitamin C may be instrumental in reducing the formation of N-nitroso compounds within the digestive tract. These substances are formed when dietary nitrate changes to nitrite, which, in turn, reacts with nitrogen-containing substances to form N-nitroso compounds, which are known to be potent cancer-forming agents.

Nitrates are present in vegetables, water and in

preserved meat products and, although evidence relating dietary intake of nitrates with cancer fail to be conclusive, there are suggestions that stomach or oesophageal cancers are the most likely of all the cancers to be influenced in this way.

Coffee

Much interest has been shown in whether or not common beverages such as coffee have long-term effects on health. A number of studies have tried to implicate coffee drinking in cancer of the breast, pancreas and bladder, but all have failed to provide more than a weak link that does not stand up to more rigorous analysis or prove positive in animal experiments.

Other Dietary Carcinogens

Certain compounds naturally present in food may act as carcinogens and some discoveries have been made in this area when isolated populations are known to eat particular foods. For instance, high rates of liver cancer appear to

be associated with the consumption of aflatoxins, produced by moulds. In tropical countries, the climate may encourage mould growth if crops such as cereals and peanuts are not carefully supervised when in storage. In Western countries such contamination is rare.

The role of food additives in cancer development is unknown, but their contribution, if any, is thought to be extremely small, perhaps less than 1 per cent. When this risk is compared to the overall estimate of the proportion of all cancers attributable to diet, which is approximately 35 per cent, it can be seen that the risk is small. Some concern has been expressed about the artificial sweetener saccharin and a link with bladder cancer that was found in some animal experiments, but the evidence for such an effect in humans has so far been inconsistent. The new sweetener aspartame has undergone rigorous tests and has been deemed safe to use.

It has been argued that the protective action of some vitamins may be via their antioxidant properties, so it seems logical to suggest that such food additives may act in the same way.

Further research will enable us to say with more certainty what the links are between diet and cancer, but it appears likely that diet will be seen as only one factor in the development of cancer.

Chapter 2

Diet after Diagnosis

Once you have been told that you have cancer, your doctors will outline your course of treatment. This may be surgery, chemotherapy (using chemicals injected into the body to destroy the cancer cells) or radiotherapy (using radiation beam treatment on the affected area to destroy the cancer cells) or a combination, but the treatment will be tailored to your own specific needs and so will be different for each person. Whatever your situation is, however, it is important that, after diagnosis, during treatment and after treatment, you maintain your body by eating a well-balanced diet.

Your body needs protein, energy, vitamins and minerals to help keep you fit during your treatment, so eat as wide a variety of foods as you can. Foods can be divided into groups of proteins, fats, carbohydrates, vitamins and minerals.

- **Proteins** are needed for tissue growth, wound healing and muscle strength. Good sources are meat, fish, poultry, cheese, eggs, milk, yoghurt and pulses, such as beans or lentils.

- **Fats and carbohydrates** are foods that give us energy. Good sources are butter, margarine, cream, oil, bread, potatoes, cereals, pasta, rice and sugary foods.

- **Vitamins and minerals** are needed in small amounts and are present in many foods (see the table on page 22 for specific vitamins and minerals).

Try and eat some foods from each group every day. If you are eating normally, this should not be problematic, but the treatments for cancer can cause eating difficulties that, although often temporary, can be distressing at the time. Usually it is your appetite that suffers and there may be times when you just do not feel like eating. Chemotherapy may cause you to feel sick, sometimes simply worries and anxieties will cause you to eat less or it may be that you lose weight because you are unable to eat your usual diet. These difficulties are not out of the ordinary and, be assured, there are ways of coping with them to enable you to eat better, which we shall come to shortly, but first let us look at what a good diet is.

What is healthy eating?

A healthy diet is one that not only provides all the energy, protein, vitamins, minerals and fibre your body needs, but also one that avoids eating an excessive amount of fat, sugar and salt. In addition to the links between diet and cancer that we saw earlier, it is known that diet can influence the development of other diseases, particularly heart disease, obesity, high blood pressure (hypertension), bowel disorders and dental decay.

Healthy eating guidelines have been produced both by advisory committees and, in some countries, by government departments. This section of the book provides guidelines for a healthy diet for you and all the family, if your appetite is good. What should perhaps be remembered is that it is your usual daily intake of food that is important — straying from the rules on holidays and special occasions is not going to undo the good of a generally healthy diet. A healthy diet is one that:

- is low in fat
- is high in fibre
- is low in sugar
- contains a wide range of vitamins and minerals
- is moderate in the amount of alcohol consumed.

Let us look at these points in more detail.

Low fat

The majority of our fat intake comes from meat products, but this does not mean that a vegetarian diet is necessarily low in fat as next on the list of sources of fat are milk, margarine, cooking oils and fats, butter, then biscuits, cakes and pastries, cheese, cream and eggs.

Of the fats in our diet some are derived from saturated fats, which are mainly of animal origin, such as butter, lard and hard margarines, some are of the polyunsaturated variety, which are those from vegetable sources, such as corn, sunflower and soya oil and the rest are monounsaturated, for example olive oil. While *saturated* fats are thought to be the most detrimental to the body because they raise the cholesterol level, it is best to cut your intake of *all* fats in the following ways:

- include meat in a low-fat diet if you wish, but make sure it is lean and cut off any visible fat
- use fish, chicken, turkey, beans and pulses as lower fat alternatives to red meat
- use a minimum of fat in cooking — grill (broil), toast or steam in preference to frying
- use low-fat dairy produce, such as skimmed (fatless) or semi-skimmed (low-fat) milk, low-fat yoghurt, low-fat or skimmed milk cheese (remember these are good sources of calcium)
- use butter or margarine sparingly or try a low-fat spread
- remember, some packaged or processed foods may be high in fat, such as cakes, pies, sausages and chocolate.

High fibre

Most of our fibre comes from vegetables, then cereals and breads and fruit. Increasing your intake of foods rich in fibre has the added advantage of also increasing your intake of vitamins and minerals. Here are some tips for making the most of both:

- choose wholemeal (wholewheat) or whole-grain cereals, such as wholemeal (whole-wheat) bread, brown rice, wholemeal (wholewheat) pasta, as these are richer in vitamins B_1, niacin, B_6 and E than the equivalent white or refined cereal products

- eat vegetables and fruit as fresh as possible for a higher vitamin content and, in fact, frozen vegetables may contain more vitamins than poorly stored fresh ones

- when cooking vegetables, steam or cook them in the minimum amount of water to reduce vitamin and mineral loss

- dried fruit is a good source of vitamins, minerals and fibre

- nuts also provide fibre but use in moderation as they are also high in fat.

Low sugar

Sugar is not only added to drinks and cooking in the home but is also to be found as an ingredient in processed foods, such as cakes, sweets, chocolate, fruit squash, fizzy drinks and unex-pected places such as savoury sauces and soups.

Eating sugar is an easy way of consuming extra energy, or calories, and often sugary foods offer little in the way of vitamins, minerals or fibre, but sugars are also present naturally in fruits, fruit juice and some vegetables and these foods provide many additional nutrients, so:

- educate your taste-buds to want less sugar by gradually reducing your intake, but remem-ber, you will gain nothing by changing to similar amounts of brown sugar or honey as these are also pure sugar

- reduce your intake of processed foods, which are high in sugar (remember that ingredients at the top of the list on the packaging are present in the largest quantity)

- use the sugar naturally present in some foods by using *them* as sweetening agents instead of sugar, such as fruit juice or dried fruit.

Vitamins and minerals

By increasing your intake of fibre-containing foods and reducing high-sugar and high-fat foods, you will automatically consume more vitamins and minerals and by eating a variety of foods you will ensure that you will be taking in a wide variety of nutrients (check with the chart on page 22 if you are interested in any particular vitamins or minerals). In addition to the vitamins and minerals already mentioned, there are a number of vitamins and trace elements required by the body. These include vitamins such as pantothenic acid and biotin and trace elements including manganese, iodine, copper and molybdenum. These tend to be present in small quantities in a wide variety of foods — another reason for making sure you do not eat the same foods all the time to the exclusion of others.

Alcohol

Be moderate about your alcohol intake as alcoholic drinks tend to be poor sources of nutrients.

Current recommendations are based on units or standard pub measures. 1 unit, or 10g, of alcohol is equal to one 4-fl oz (125-ml) glass of wine, one 2-fl oz (60-ml) glass of sherry or port or ½ pint (275ml) of beer or cider, but bear in mind that strong beer or strong lager contains a higher percentage of alcohol. The recommended limits for alcohol consumption are that:

- women should not exceed 14 units per week
- men should not exceed 21 units per week.

Why not try some of the low-alcohol wines or beers now widely available.

Overweight

If you are overweight it may be sensible to lose some weight unless you are currently having treatment, in which case, check first with your doctor.

Vitamins and Minerals

Vitamin	Sources
Vitamin C (ascorbic acid) Necessary for the formation of connective tissue and therefore wound healing.	Fruit and fruit juices, especially blackcurrants, citrus fruits, vegetables, including green leafy vegetables, Brussels sprouts and cauliflower, liver and kidney, potatoes.
Vitamin B$_1$ (thiamin) Necessary to enable the body to use carbohydrates efficiently.	Wholegrains, such as wheat, millet and brown rice, pulses, such as beans and lentils, fruit and vegetables and pork, beef, fish, milk and eggs.
Vitamin B$_2$ (riboflavin) Necessary for the use of oxygen by the cells.	Liver, milk, eggs, green vegetables, yeast and meat extracts.

Vitamin	Sources
Nicotinic acid (niacin) Necessary for the use of oxygen by the cells.	Liver, kidney, beef, mutton, pork, fish, brewer's yeast and meat extracts, and moderate sources include pulses, nuts, dried fruits and oatmeal.
Vitamin B$_6$ Necessary for functioning of numerous enzymes.	Liver, wholegrain cereals, peanuts and bananas. Most foods contain moderate amounts.
Folate Necessary for formation of red blood cells.	Liver, spinach, broccoli tops, kidney, pulses, and moderate sources include wholemeal (wholewheat) bread, and eggs and fruit, such as oranges, and bananas.
Vitamin B$_{12}$ Necessary for DNA formation and therefore required by all cells.	Egg yolks, cheese, and a moderate source is milk. Not present in any plants.
Vitamin A (retinol) Necessary for formation of pigment rhodopsin in eye. Necessary for formation of cells especially in the eyes, skin and lungs.	Oily fish and halibut and cod liver oil, liver, butter, margarine, eggs, milk and cheese are sources of retinol, and carrots, leafy vegetables and apricots are sources of β-carotene.
Vitamin D (cholecalciferol) Necessary for calcium and phosphate regulation in body.	Liver oils of fish, oily fish, eggs, butter, milk, margarine, and manufactured by body in response to sunlight.
Vitamin E (tocopherols) Helps to protect the cell membrane.	Vegetable oils including wheatgerm, sunflower and safflower, and moderate sources are eggs, butter, wholemeal cereals and broccoli.

Mineral	Sources
Calcium Necessary for strong bones and teeth, nerve function, muscle action and blood clotting.	Milk and milk products, and moderate sources are nuts, pulses, sardines and pilchards.
Iron Necessary for haemoglobin formation in red blood cells.	Liver, red meat, eggs, fish and green leafy vegetables.
Zinc Necessary for cell metabolism, growth and wound healing.	Meat, wholegrain cereals, pulses and nuts.
Magnesium Necessary for cell metabolism.	Cereals and vegetables.
Selenium Component of enzyme glutathione peroxidase, which prevents oxidative damage of cells.	Fish, meat and cereals.

Eating difficulties during your treatment

If you are experiencing any of the eating difficulties described earlier in the chapter the following suggestions may help you to overcome them.

In general, if you are not eating very well, try to have small meals or snacks more often, spreading your food intake more evenly through the day instead of keeping to three meals a day. Make use of convenience foods and nourishing drinks such as those listed on page 28.

If you have not been eating well for a long time, you may not be taking in enough vitamins in food form and may therefore need to take a multivitamin supplement. Ask your doctor or dietitian for advice.

It may be that your illness or the treatment for it has caused your specific eating difficulties. Some of the most common problems and practical ways to cope with these are given below.

Lost your appetite?

This is a very common problem and often appetite tends to come and go in cycles. It is important, then, to make the most of the times when you *do* feel like eating. When you do not feel like eating, try to tempt the appetite by eating the foods you like, even if these are foods like chocolate bars, cakes or fizzy drinks. Try, too, eating small amounts of food at a time as a little and often is an easier way of eating when your appetite is poor than facing a whole plate of food. Have small meals, with snacks and nourishing drinks in between.

Some ideas for small, quick and easy meals or snacks are:

- sandwiches, plain or toasted
- cereals with milk and sugar
- tinned snacks, such as spaghetti, baked beans or macaroni cheese
- jacket potatoes, either plain or with cheese or butter.

For dessert you could try:

- yoghurts
- fromage frais
- crème caramel (readymade or home-made, see page 63 for recipe)

- instant or tinned (canned) puddings
- milk puddings

You could also try some of the instant nourishing drinks available from most chemists that are meals in themselves. Similar drinks are also available on prescription in the UK so talk to your doctor about this. There is more information about these drinks at the end of this chapter and you may also like to try some of the home-made nourishing drink recipes given on pages 78-89.

A very pleasant way of encouraging your appetite is to try an aperitif, as a small drink, such as sherry or brandy, taken about half an hour before meals can help to stimulate your desire for food. If you are on any medication, though, check with your doctor or pharmacist first that you can take alcohol without any side effects.

Feeling full too soon?

If you have not got much of an appetite, you may find that you feel full quickly. This is another reason why small, frequent meals or snacks may suit you better. You may find the following ideas helpful, too:

- avoid greasy, fried food or rich sauces as these foods can make you feel full quickly
- If you like having drinks — soft drinks, tea or coffee and so on — have them half an hour before or after meals otherwise the fluid may fill you up to the extent where you cannot eat much before feeling you cannot eat any more.

Feeling sick?

Hopefully any nausea you feel will only be temporary, but, however long it lasts, it is important to try to eat during this time. Try the following:

- avoid unpleasant smells or smells of food cooking, as smells, however pleasant they seem any other time, often make people feel more sick when they are nauseous
- if possible, have someone else prepare food for you
- cold foods and drinks may be better as they don't have such a strong smell
- avoid hot, spicy or greasy foods
- eat something dry such as toast, or plain biscuits
- keep meals fairly dry and have drinks a little after meals
- try sipping a fizzy drink such as soda water or dry ginger ale.

Ask your doctor to prescribe something if your sickness remains a problem.

Is chewing or swallowing difficult?

If you are having problems chewing or swallowing normally or you have a sore mouth or throat, then you may need a soft or puréed diet. If so, see your dietitian or doctor for specific help but here are a few ideas:

- choose soft foods, (see recipes marked as suitable for chewing and swallowing difficulties)
- Purée food in a blender if necessary — you can purée most foods from the family menu, for example, meat, chicken, vegetables — but the food looks and tastes better if the parts of the meal are puréed separately rather than all together and read the instruction booklet for your blender carefully (most blenders also come with recipe booklets that will give you more ideas for meals)
- use extra butter, sauces and gravies to soften foods
- avoid rough, coarse or very dry foods
- have plenty of nourishing drinks (see pages 78-89 for recipes)
- commercially available baby foods may be useful although extra seasoning may be necessary.

Here are some ideas for soft main courses:

- tinned or home-made soup (see pages 35-36 for recipes)
- minced or puréed roast meat and gravy
- shepherd's pie
- lasagne
- cannelloni (see page 43 for recipe)
- soft poached fish in sauce
- salmon mousse (see page 40 for recipe)
- omelette or scrambled egg (see page 52 for recipe)
- savoury baked egg custard
- creamed chicken or ham
- corned beef hash (see page 42 for recipe)
- cheese pudding (see page 54 for recipe).

Good soft desserts include:

- mousse (see page 61 for recipe)
- egg custard (see page 60 for recipe)
- crème caramel (see page 63 for recipe)
- milk puddings
- fruit whisk (see page 57 for recipe)
- soufflés (see page 71 for recipe)
- sorbets
- ice-cream (see page 85 for recipe)
- yoghurts
- fromage frais
- custard
- tinned fruit
- tinned or instant puddings.

Has your sense of taste changed?

You may find that your food tastes strange or that you've lost your sense of taste. This is usually a temporary change, but here are a few ideas to help you make your food more palatable while the sensation lasts:

- use more or stronger seasonings to enhance the flavour of food, for example, herbs, spices, garlic or sauces
- marinate foods such as meat, fish or chicken to give them a richer flavour
- concentrate on foods that still taste good
- try having sharp drinks such as fruit juices or suck sweets (candies) to help eliminate any bad taste.

Lost weight?

If you have had problems eating for some time, it may be that you have lost or are losing weight. It is not a good idea to lose too much weight before or during your treatment so if you are losing weight or have lost weight then you should see a dietitian for specific advice. In the meantime, though the following ideas might help:

- eat small, frequent meals, with snacks or nourishing drinks in between
- try to add extra protein and calories to your diet without increasing the quantity of food you are eating by:
  - using fortified milk (see page 78 for recipe) in place of ordinary milk
  - using milk to make up packet or condensed soups, jellies and so on
  - adding extra butter to vegetables, pasta and bread or toast
  - using cream or yoghurt in sauces
  - adding cream to your cereal or to puddings/desserts
- use some of the commercially available protein and energy supplements (see below)
- have extra nourishing drinks either commercial (see page 28) or home-made (see pages 78-89 for recipes).

Commercially available nutritional supplements

Before using any of these supplements *please* seek advice from your doctor or dietitian on the type and quantity of supplement needed in your particular circumstances as these products should only be used under medical and/or dietetic supervision.

Commercially available nourishing drinks

These are specially formulated drinks that can be used as meal replacements or as supplementary drinks between meals. They are nutritionally complete, that is, they contain the whole range of nutrients. Some are powders that you make up with milk or water and some examples of these in the UK are Build Up (Nestlé) or Complan (Glaxo), in the USA, Meritene (Sandoz), Forta Shake (Abbott/Ross) and in Australia, Ensure (Abbott/Ross).

Liquid nutritional drinks that you do not need to add anything to are also available. Examples of these in the UK are Fortisip (Cow & Gate), Ensure (Abbott/Ross) and Fresubin (Fresenius) and in Australia and the USA, Ensure and Ensure Plus (Abbott/Ross). All of these products come in a wide range of flavours, both savoury and sweet. Some are available on prescription from your doctor, but ask your doctor or dietitian anyway for advice on the products available.

Commercially available energy supplements

These are available as powders or liquids that can be added to food or drink.

The glucose polymer powders are white powders that look like glucose but do not taste sweet and can be added to most drinks or incorporated into recipes to increase their energy content. Some brand names that you will see include Maxijul (Scientific Hospital Supplies) and Polycal (Cow & Gate) in the UK. Polycose (Abbott/Ross) is available in the UK, Australia and the USA.

You can also get glucose drinks and these come in a range of flavours so that they can be mixed with milk shakes, water, fruit juices or fizzy drinks. They can also be added to puddings or made into jellies or ice lollies. Brand names of this type of energy supplement include Fortical (Cow & Gate), Hycal (Beechams) and Maxijul (Scientific Hospital Supplies), in the UK. Polycose (Abbott/Ross) and Forta Drink (Abbott/Ross) in the USA.

Most of these products are available in the UK on prescription from your doctor.

Commercially available protein supplements

There are powdered protein supplements available that can be added to drinks or food such as soups and puddings. Examples of these products include Maxipro (Scientific Hospital Supplies) and Casilan (Glaxo). These, too, are available in the UK on prescription from your doctor. Promod (Abbott/Ross) is available in the UK, Australia and the USA.

New commercial nutritional products appear regularly so it is important to ask your dietitian for up-to-date information.

Chapter 3

Complementary Dietary Therapies

This phrase refers to any unusual or unconventional modifications to a normal diet that are claimed to be of benefit to patients with cancer. They are normally recommended in conjunction with conventional anti-cancer therapies such as chemotherapy or radiotherapy, most derive from the United States of America or the Far East and are very popular with cancer patients. Examples of such complementary diets are:

- the Bristol Diet, which originates from the Bristol Cancer Help Centre in the UK
- macrobiotics, which originated in Japan but has been much publicized by the Kushi Institute in the USA
- the Gerson Therapy, a very strict therapy now practised at the Gerson Therapy Centre in Mexico.

These dietary therapies claim to benefit the cancer patient by increasing well-being, reducing symptoms and increasing health. As these regimes are so popular, it is worth considering them in a little more detail.

The Bristol Diet

The Bristol Diet is not an isolated dietary regime but just one part of a programme of activities including visualization, relaxation and so on. The diet is low-fat, low-sugar and vegan and the general guidelines are as follows:

- **foods allowed**: fresh vegetables, organically grown if possible; wholegrain cereals, such as brown rice, wheat, barley, rye, maize, oats, buckwheat; pulses, nuts, tofu, soya milk, goat's milk yoghurt, wholemeal (wholewheat) pasta, 100 per cent wholemeal (wholewheat) bread, fresh fruit, herbs and spices, spring water, herb tea, fresh fruit and vegetable juices, honey, molasses and ghee (clarified butter)

- **foods to avoid**: meat, fish, eggs, cheese, milk, frozen or tinned fruit or vegetables, white bread, refined cereals, tea, coffee, fizzy drinks, sugar or sugary foods, jams and marmalades, shop-bought cakes and biscuits, ice-cream, all commercially produced foods.

The Bristol regime also includes large doses of vitamin and mineral supplements.

A study reported in *The Lancet*, September 1990, found that women with breast cancer who attended the Bristol Cancer Help Centre (between 1986 and 1988) while receiving conventional therapy did significantly worse than those women receiving conventional therapy alone. This, naturally, has led both the Bristol Centre and the medical profession to question the suitability of this treatment for cancer patients, although there is now doubt as to whether the two groups were actually comparable. If you are interested in the Bristol Centre regimes, then we suggest that you discuss the matter with the doctor responsible for your treatment.

Macrobiotics

One important thing to bear in mind with macrobiotics is that it is not just a diet, but a philosophy of life. The dietary concepts within the philosophy have been used in 'natural healing' for hundreds of years. Foods are grouped under the headings Yin and Yang. This is a complex system of classification based on the composition of the food, how it is grown, when it is grown and so on. Any illness, including cancer, can also be classified as either Yin or Yang. According to whether a person's overall condition is more Yin or Yang, the proportion of Yin and Yang foods in the diet will be altered to re-attain balance within the body — a balanced body

being a healthy body. The diet, therefore, needs to be skilfully calculated for each individual, but here are some of the basic principles:

● it is vegan (with the very occasional inclusion of white meat or fish)

● 50 per cent of each meal should consist of cereals, such as wholemeal (wholewheat) bread, rice, corn and so on

● large quantities of raw vegetables are recommended

● it is low-salt

● it is low-fat.

Gerson Therapy

The Gerson Therapy is an extremely strict dietary regime. It is the only regime that claims to 'cure' cancer rather than increase well-being and reduce symptoms. Usually, followers of the Gerson Therapy are required to give up conventional treatments, that is, chemotherapy or radiotherapy.

The therapy consists of a high-potassium, low-sodium, vegan-type diet with little fat and minimal quantities of animal protein. The juices of raw fruits, vegetables and of raw liver are recommended. Coffee enemas are also recommended regularly on this regime.

For more detailed information on these dietary therapies you will find sources given in the reading list on page 142.

Complementary dietary therapies such as

these three do seem to be of benefit to some cancer patients. This benefit may be associated with the positive attitude that these therapies inspire and the fact that they provide one way for patients to have some kind of control over their treatment. Most dietary regimes are closely linked with other holistic therapies such as relaxation, visualization or therapeutic massage and the combination of techniques certainly increases the sense of well-being in those who try them. It is unlikely that the diets *alone* have any real medical benefit and, as yet, there is little research into such diets.

Many patients following such complementary regimes also have eating difficulties such as loss of appetite and may be losing weight. Complementary diets tend to be high in bulk and low in energy, difficult to prepare and costly, and eating large amounts of high bulk food is very difficult if appetite is poor. Following such regimes often leads to weight loss and, hence, deterioration in nutritional status. The most important point to emphasize, however, is that any diet, 'normal' or 'complementary', needs to provide a good, well-balanced intake of food so as to maintain the body in a state of good nutrition. For this reason, patients following, or contemplating following, any complementary dietary regimen should seek advice from a dietitian.

Like all therapies, it is a matter of individual choice, but make sure that in exercising that right you take account of *all* the advantages and disadvantages of a dietary therapy before coming to a decision. If you wish, it is sometimes possible to accommodate particular aspects of such diets into a conventionally planned nutritional programme, providing it does not harm you and does not conflict with treatment. The dietitian is the best person to give advice on these matters so be sure to consult him or her carefully.

Part 2

Recipes for Those with Eating Difficulties

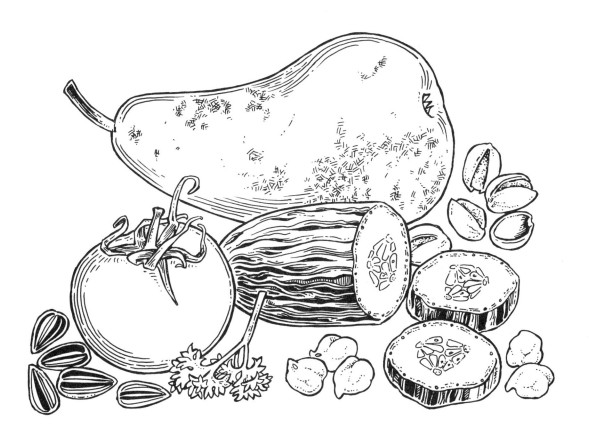

Chapter 4

Starters

Lettuce Soup

This dish is suitable for those with chewing and swallowing difficulties.

Imperial/metric	Serves 4	American
1 oz (30g)	butter	2tbs
1	medium onion, chopped	1
1	medium potato, chopped	1
1	lettuce, washed	1
1½ pts (850ml)	milk	3¾ cups
½ pt (285ml)	chicken stock	1⅓ cups
1 pinch	dill	1 pinch
	seasoning to taste	
¼ pt (140ml)	single cream/light cream	⅔ cup
2 tbs	chives, snipped, to garnish	2 tbs

1. Melt the butter and sauté the onion and potato until soft.

2. Stir in the lettuce and toss with the onion and potato mixture.

3. Add the milk, stock, dill and seasoning.

4. Bring to the boil, then cover and simmer for 10-15 minutes.

5. Let it cool slightly.

6. Liquidize (blend) the soup.

7. Add the cream just before serving.

8. Garnish with the snipped chives and serve.

CAN BE FROZEN

Chilled Cream of Broccoli Soup

This is a high energy dish and suitable for those with chewing and swallowing difficulties and taste changes.

Imperial/metric	Serves 4	American
1¼ pts (710ml)	chicken stock	3¼ cups
1 lb (455g)	frozen broccoli, defrosted and sliced	1 lb
1	stick/stalk celery, sliced	1
1	small onion, sliced	1
	salt	
	freshly ground black pepper	
7 fl oz (200ml)	double/heavy cream	¾ cup

1. Pour the stock into a saucepan. Add the broccoli, celery and onion.
2. Bring to the boil, then cover, reduce the heat and simmer for 20 minutes.

3. Pour the soup into a liquidizer (blender), blend until smooth and season with salt and pepper. Chill for 3 hours.
4. Before serving, stir the cream into the soup.

Brie and Courgette Soup

This is a high energy soup suitable for those with chewing and swallowing difficulties.

Imperial/metric	Serves 4	American
¾ lb (340g)	courgettes/zucchini, sliced	2 cups
6 oz (170g)	potato, peeled and diced	1 cup
1 tbs	sunflower oil	1 tbs
	salt to taste	
4 oz (115g)	soft, ripe Brie, no rind, diced	½ cup
	freshly ground black pepper	
2 fl oz (60ml)	double/heavy cream	¼ cup

1. Put the courgette (zucchini) slices in a pan with the potatoes, oil and salt, cover with water, stir and bring to the boil. Simmer for 15-20 minutes, then let cool slightly.
2. Remove the courgettes (zucchini) and potatoes to a liquidizer (blender), leaving the liquid. Liquidize (blend) with the Brie and ½ pt (285ml/1⅓ cups) of the cooking liquid. Pour the rest of the liquid into a jug.
3. Return the soup to the pan, adding another ¼ pt (140ml/⅔ cup) of the reserved cooking liquid. Bring the soup to the boil slowly, stirring constantly. Add more cooking water if necessary.
4. Add salt and freshly ground black pepper to taste.
5. Pour into serving bowls and finish with a swirl of cream.

Smoked Mackerel Pâté

This dish is suitable for those with chewing and swallowing difficulties and taste changes.

Imperial/metric	Serves 4	American
½ lb (225g)	smoked mackerel fillets, cooked	½ lb
4 oz (115g)	curd/ricotta cheese	½ cup
4 oz (115g)	cottage/pot cheese	½ cup
	juice of 1 lemon	
	freshly ground black pepper	
1 tsp	fresh parsley, finely chopped	1 tsp

1. Remove the skin from the fish and take care to remove all bones.
2. Put the fish in a liquidizer (blender) with the cheeses, lemon juice, black pepper and parsley.
3. Liquidize (blend) the mixture until it is smooth.
4. Press the pâté into a greased container and chill well prior to serving.

Tuna Pâté

This is a high energy dish and is suitable for those with chewing and swallowing difficulties and taste changes.

Imperial/metric	Serves 4	American
6 oz (170g)	butter	¾ cup
1 × 7 oz (200g)	tin/can tuna, drained	1 × 7 oz
2 tbs	lemon juice	2 tbs
2 tbs	vegetable oil	2 tbs
2 tbs	brandy	2 tbs
1	clove garlic, crushed/minced	1
1 tbs	parsley, chopped	1 tbs
1	small onion, finely chopped	1
	salt	
	freshly ground black pepper	

1. Melt the butter in a saucepan.
2. Mash the tuna with the lemon juice, oil and brandy.

3. Add the melted butter, garlic, parsley, onion and season to taste. Blend well.

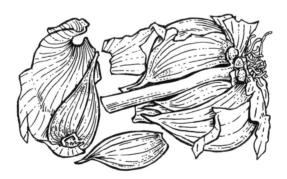

Smoked Oyster Pâté

This is a high energy recipe. It is suitable for those with chewing and swallowing difficulties and for taste changes.

Imperial/metric	Serves 4	American
5 fl oz (140ml)	hot water	⅔ cup
1	chicken stock cube	1
2 tsp	gelatine	2 tsp
2 × 3½ oz (105g)	tins/cans smoked oysters, drained and chopped	2 × 3½ oz
3	shallots or chives, chopped	3
4 fl oz (120ml)	sour cream	½ cup
3 fl oz (90ml)	mayonnaise	⅓ cup
	salt	
	freshly ground black pepper	
	Topping	
3 tbs	mayonnaise	3 tbs
3	shallots, chopped	3
2 tbs	fresh parsley, chopped	2 tbs

1. Put the hot water, stock cube and gelatine in a liquidizer (blender) and blend for approximately 30 seconds.

2. Add the oysters, shallots or chives, sour cream, mayonnaise, salt and pepper and blend until smooth. Press the mixture into a pâté dish and chill in the refrigerator until set.

3. For the topping, blend together the mayonnaise, shallots and parsley. Pour it over the pâté and chill until firm.

Salmon Mousse

This is a high energy recipe and suitable for those with chewing and swallowing problems.

Imperial/metric	Serves 4	American
1½ tbs	gelatine	1½ tbs
3 fl oz (90ml)	cold water	⅓ cup
7 fl oz (200ml)	chicken stock, hot	¾ cup
2 × 7 oz (200g)	tins/cans salmon, drained	2 × 7 oz
2 tbs	tomato purée/paste	2 tbs
2 tbs	vinegar	2 tbs
1 tbs	Worcestershire sauce	1 tbs
5 fl oz (140ml)	mayonnaise	⅔ cup
	salt	
	freshly ground black pepper	
7 fl oz (200ml)	double/heavy cream	¾ cup
2	egg whites (optional)	2

1. Soak the gelatine in the cold water and stir the mixture into the hot stock to dissolve the granules.

2. Put the salmon, stock, tomato purée (paste), vinegar, Worcestershire sauce, mayonnaise, salt and pepper into a liquidizer (blender) and blend until smooth.

3. Whip the cream and fold into the salmon mixture when it is just beginning to set.

4. If the egg whites are used, beat them until they are stiff and then fold them into the salmon mixture.

5. Divide the mousse into 4 ramekins and chill for 2 hours before serving.

Mushroom Spread

This is good as a spread on Melba toast or as a dip for crudités and as a nourishing snack. The recipe is suitable for those with chewing and swallowing difficulties and taste changes.

Imperial/metric	*Serves 4*	American
8 oz (225g)	mushrooms, chopped	3 cups
½ oz (15g)	onion, chopped	1 tbs
4 oz (115g)	butter	½ cup
3 oz (85g)	soft, full-fat cream cheese	6 tbs
	dash of Worcestershire sauce	
	dash of lemon juice	
	salt and pepper to taste	

1. Fry the mushrooms and onion in the butter for 2-3 minutes.

2. Put the mixture into a liquidizer (blender) with the cheese, Worcestershire sauce, lemon juice and salt and pepper and blend together until smooth.

3. Press into a pâté dish and chill in the refrigerator until set.

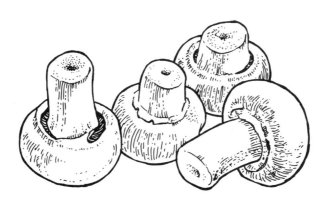

Chapter 5

Main Courses

Corned Beef Hash

This dish is suitable for those with chewing and swallowing difficulties.

Imperial/metric	Serves 4	American
1 × 12 oz (340g)	tin/can corned beef	1 × 12 oz
1	onion, peeled and finely chopped	1
12 oz (340g)	potato, peeled and diced	2 cups
½	stock/bouillon cube	½
¼ pt (140ml)	water	⅔ cup
	salt	
	freshly ground black pepper	
1 dsp	Worcestershire sauce	2 tsp

1. Put all the ingredients in a saucepan, crumble in the stock (bouillon) cube, and bring to the boil. Cover, reduce the heat and simmer for ¾-1 hour until the potatoes are soft.

CAN BE FROZEN

Microwave Cannelloni

This dish is suitable for those with chewing and swallowing difficulties.

Imperial/metric	Serves 4	American
1½ oz (45g)	butter or margarine	2½ tbs
1 oz (30g)	plain/all-purpose flour	2 tbs
¾ pt (425ml)	milk	2 cups
	salt and pepper to taste	
2 oz (55g)	cheese, grated	½ cup
1	onion, finely chopped	1
1 clove	garlic, crushed/minced	1 clove
1 tsp	dried basil	1 tsp
	pinch nutmeg	
8 oz (225g)	minced/ground beef	½ lb
2 oz (55g)	bacon, chopped	2 slices
2 heaped tsp	tomato purée/paste	2 heaped tsp
1 × 8 oz (225g)	tin/can tomatoes	1 × 8 oz
8	pasta cannelloni tubes	8

1. Melt the butter or margarine.

2. Blend in the flour and cook gently for a minute.

3. Gradually add in the milk and stir quickly to combine and continue stirring until the sauce thickens.

4. Add salt and pepper to taste and ⅔ of the cheese.

5. Put the onion, garlic, basil and nutmeg in a microwave bowl and cook on high for 2-3 minutes.

6. Add the beef, bacon, tomato purée (paste) and tomatoes and season to taste.

7. Cover and cook on high for 5 minutes, stirring the mixture half-way through cooking, then allow to cool.

8. Stuff the cannelloni tubes with the beef mixture using a spoon and place them in a microwave dish.

9. Cover the tubes with the cheese sauce and cook on high for 10 minutes.

10. Sprinkle the dish with the reserved cheese and brown under the grill (broiler).

<u>CAN BE FROZEN</u>

Boboke

This dish is suitable for those experiencing taste changes.

Imperial/metric	Serves 4	American
1 slice	white bread	1 slice
¼ pt (140ml)	milk	⅔ cup
2	medium onions, chopped	2
1 tbs	curry powder	1 tbs
	pinch of salt	
3	medium tomatoes, chopped	3
	pinch of sugar	
½ oz (15g)	butter	1 tbs
1	egg	1
1 lb (455g)	minced/ground beef	1 lb
½ tbs	chutney	½ tbs

1. Soak the bread in the milk and then mash it with a fork.

2. Fry one onion in half the butter and add the curry powder and salt.

3. Mix the second onion with the tomatoes and sprinkle with salt and sugar to taste.

4. Melt the remaining butter in a saucepan and gently cook the onion and tomato mixture.

5. Mix the egg, beef, onion and tomato mixture, curried onion and chutney together and pour into a greased pie dish.

6. Bake in a moderate oven at 350°F/180°C (Gas Mark 4) for 1½ hours.

CAN BE FROZEN

Chicken Valentine

This is a high energy dish and is suitable for those experiencing taste changes.

Imperial/metric	Serves 4	American
4	chicken breasts	4
4 oz (115g)	butter	1 stick
4 oz (115g)	plain/all-purpose flour	1 cup
1 glass (140ml)	white wine	⅔ cup
½ pt (285ml)	milk	1⅓ cups
	salt and pepper to taste	
1	small onion, chopped	1
1 × 14 oz (395g)	tin/can asparagus, trimmed and finely chopped	1 × 14 oz
1 oz (30g)	butter	2 tbs
1 small (125g) carton	natural/plain yoghurt	1 small (125g) carton
	sprigs of fresh parsley to garnish	

1. Roast the chicken breasts, wrapped in foil, in a 350°F/180°C (Gas Mark 4) oven for 25 minutes. Meanwhile, make the sauce as follows.
2. Melt the butter in a pan and whisk in the flour.
3. Add the wine and half the milk slowly until the sauce is fluid, then season to taste.
4. Sauté the onion in the butter until it is transparent, then strain and add to the sauce.
5. Add the asparagus to the sauce.

6. Add the rest of the milk, mixing well so the sauce has a creamy consistency, and simmer gently for approximately 5-10 minutes until the asparagus is tender.
7. Add a tbs of the yoghurt to the sauce and stir in.
8. Place one chicken breast on each plate and pour the sauce over it. Pour a spoonful of yoghurt over the top of that and garnish with parsley.

Coronation Chicken

This is a high energy dish and is suitable for those experiencing taste changes.

Imperial/metric	Serves 4	American
6 oz (170g)	mushrooms, sliced	3 cups
1 oz (30g)	butter	2 tbs
1	large onion, chopped	1
1 lb (455g)	tomatoes, fresh or tinned/canned, chopped	1 lb
1 packet	instant chicken soup powder (to serve 1)	1 packet
⅓ pt (200ml)	chicken stock	¾ cup
1 × 6 oz (170ml)	tin/can sterilized cream	1 × 6 oz
4	medium chicken breasts	4
2 oz (50g)	cheese, grated	½ cup

1. Cook the mushrooms in the butter, then remove with a slotted spoon and keep to one side.
2. Add the onion, tomatoes and chicken soup powder to the pan and stir together well.
3. Add the stock and bring to the boil.
4. Add the cream and cook gently for 5 minutes.

5. Put the chicken pieces in an ovenproof dish, sprinkle the reserved mushrooms over the chicken, pour the onion and tomato sauce over the top and sprinkle with the cheese.
6. Cook in fairly hot oven, 400°F/200°C (Gas Mark 6) for 30 minutes.

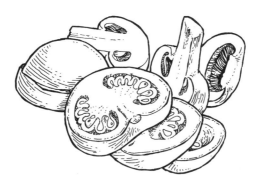

Broccoli, Chicken and Cheese Bake

This is a high energy dish and is suitable for those experiencing taste changes.

Imperial/metric	Serves 5-6	American
1½ lb (680g)	broccoli	1½ lb
3 lb (1360g)	chicken, cooked, skinned and sliced	3 lb
2 × 10 oz (285g)	tins/cans condensed chicken or mushroom soup	2 × 10 oz
4 tbs	mayonnaise	4 tbs
1 tsp	lemon juice	1 tsp
2 tsp	curry powder	2 tsp
6 oz (170g)	fresh white breadcrumbs	3 cups
4 oz (115g)	cheese, grated	1 cup
1 oz (30g)	margarine	2 tbs

1. Trim and lightly cook the broccoli.
2. Put the broccoli in the bottom of a slightly greased ovenproof dish.
3. Cover with layers of the chicken.
4. Mix the soup, mayonnaise, lemon juice and curry powder together and pour the mixture over the chicken layer.

5. Mix the breadcrumbs and cheese together and sprinkle over the soup mixture.
6. Dot the top with small pieces of margarine.
7. Bake in a moderately hot oven, 375°F/190°C (Gas Mark 5), for 45 minutes.

Chicken Liver Risotto

This dish is suitable for those experiencing taste changes.

Imperial/metric	Serves 4	American
6	chicken livers, cut into small slices	6
3 oz (85g)	onion, chopped	½ cup
2 oz (55g)	butter	¼ cup
2 oz (55g)	mushrooms, sliced	1 cup
	pinch salt	
1 tsp	white wine	1 tsp
6 oz (170g)	white rice	¾ cup
¾ pt (425ml)	chicken stock	1½ cups
2 tbs	fresh parsley, chopped	2 tbs
2 oz (55g)	parmesan cheese, grated	½ cup

1. Sauté the livers and onion gently in the butter in a large, heavy-bottomed saucepan until tender.
2. Add the mushrooms, salt, white wine, rice and stock, bring to the boil and stir once.

3. Cover the pan tightly and simmer for 15 minutes.
4. Sprinkle the top with the parsley and cheese just before serving.

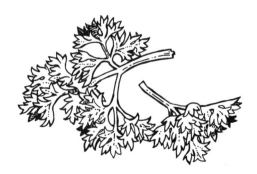

Sweet and Sour Fish

Serve this dish with rice for a truly oriental flavour. It is suitable for those experiencing taste changes.

Imperial/metric	Serves 4	American
2 tbs	sugar	2 tbs
5 tbs	cider or wine vinegar	5 tbs
8 tbs	pineapple juice	8 tbs
2 tbs	tomato purée/paste	2 tbs
1 tbs	cornflour/cornstarch	1 tbs
	salt and freshly ground black pepper	
1 tbs	sunflower oil	1 tbs
1	medium onion, chopped	1
1	sweet/red pepper, chopped	1
4 oz (115g)	tinned/canned pineapple, chopped	1 cup
1½ lb (680g)	white fish fillets, e.g. haddock	1½ lb

1. Pre-heat the oven to 350°F/180°C (Gas Mark 4).

2. Mix the sugar, vinegar, pineapple juice and tomato purée (paste) together and blend with the cornflour (cornstarch) to a smooth consistency. Add salt and pepper.

3. Heat the sunflower oil in a pan, add the onion and pepper and fry gently for 5 minutes, stirring occasionally. Add the pineapple.

4. Add the sauce and gently bring to the boil, stirring constantly.

5. Cook on a low heat for 2 minutes until it is thick. (Freeze it at this point if desired.)

6. Put the fish fillets in a large, ovenproof dish, then pour the sauce over them.

7. Place in the oven and bake for 30-40 minutes or until the fish is cooked.

CAN BE FROZEN

Fluffy Tuna Flan

This dish is suitable for those with chewing and swallowing difficulties and taste changes.

Imperial/metric	Serves 4	American
6 oz (170g)	ready-made shortcrust pastry	6 oz
1 packet	savoury white sauce mix	1 packet
1 × 7 oz (200g)	tin/can tuna, drained	1 × 7 oz
	grated rind of ½ lemon	
¼ tsp	mustard	¼ tsp
	seasoning to taste	
	2 eggs, separated	

1. Line a 9-in (23-cm) flan tin (pan) with the pastry, fill with baking or dried beans and bake in a fairly hot oven, 400°F/200°C (Gas Mark 6), for 10 minutes.
2. Make the white sauce as instructed on the packet.
3. Flake the tuna into the sauce and add the lemon rind, mustard, seasoning and egg yolks. Mix well.

4. Whisk the egg whites until stiff and gently fold them into the sauce and tuna mixture.
5. Turn this mixture into the pastry case and bake for 20-25 minutes in a fairly hot oven, 400°F/200°C (Gas Mark 6), until the filling is well risen and golden brown.

Fish and Cheese Crumble

This dish is suitable for those with chewing and swallowing difficulties.

Imperial/metric	Serves 4	American
1 lb (455g)	haddock or cod fillet	1 lb
¼ pt (140ml)	milk	⅔ cup
1	egg yolk, beaten	1
1 tsp	fresh parsley, chopped	1 tsp
	salt and pepper to taste	
2	large tomatoes, skinned and sliced	2
1½ oz (45g)	margarine	3 tbs
4 oz (115g)	plain/all-purpose flour	1 cup
2 oz (55g)	cheese, grated	½ cup
	pinch of cayenne pepper	

1. Poach the fish by gently simmering it in the milk for about 10 minutes, covering the pan. It is done when the fish flakes easily. Drain, reserving the milk.

2. Flake the fish, removing any bones.

3. Pour the reserved milk into a bowl, add the egg yolk, parsley, salt and pepper and mix together well.

4. Put the fish into a greased 1½ pt (850ml/quart) baking dish.

5. Pour the milk mixture over the fish and arrange the tomatoes, overlapping the slices, on top.

6. Make the topping by rubbing 1 oz (30g/2 tbs) of the margarine into the flour until it resembles breadcrumbs.

7. Stir in the cheese, cayenne pepper and a little salt into the topping mix.

8. Sprinkle the topping mixture evenly over the tomato layer.

9. Dot the remaining margarine over the topping.

10. Bake in a moderate oven, 350°F/180°C (Gas Mark 4), for 35 minutes.

11. Increase the heat to moderately hot, 375°F/190°C (Gas Mark 5), for 10 minutes until the topping has turned golden brown.

Savoury Omelette

This dish is suitable for those with chewing and swallowing difficulties and taste changes.

Imperial/metric	Serves 4	American
2	small potatoes, diced	2
2 tbs	cooking oil	2 tbs
1	leek, chopped	1
4 oz (115g)	bacon, chopped	4 slices
2 oz (55g)	mushrooms, chopped	¾ cup
4	large/extra large eggs	4
	salt and pepper to taste	

1. Cook the potatoes gently in the oil in an omelette or frying pan (skillet) for about 10 minutes.
2. Add the leek, bacon and mushrooms and cook gently for a further 10 minutes.
3. Break the eggs into a bowl, season with salt and pepper and beat well.

4. Pour the eggs over the cooked vegetables in the pan and cook over a low heat until the bottom is cooked.
5. Place the pan under the grill (broiler) and continue to cook until the omelette is set and just turning golden brown.

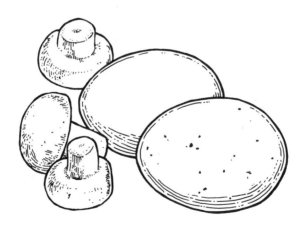

Quiche Lorraine

This is a high energy dish and is suitable for those with chewing and swallowing difficulties and taste changes.

Imperial/metric	*Serves 4*	American
8 oz (225g)	plain/all-purpose flour	2 cups
	pinch salt	
2 oz (55g)	margarine	¼ cup
1	egg yolk	1
2 tbs	cold water	2 tbs
½ tsp	lemon juice	½ tsp
	Filling	
6 oz (170g)	bacon, chopped	1½ cups
1 oz (30g) margarine	margarine	2 tbs
1 oz (30g)	spring onions/scallions, chopped	⅔ cup
2	eggs	2
⅓ pt (200ml)	milk	¾ cup
4 tbs	single/light cream	4 tbs
2 oz (55g)	cheese, grated	½ cup
	salt and pepper to taste	

1. Sift the flour and salt into a bowl.

2. Cut the margarine into small pieces and rub into the flour until fine.

3. Beat the egg yolk with the cold water and lemon juice, add gradually to the flour mixture and mix to form a soft dough.

4. Now prepare the filling. Cook the bacon gently in the margarine.

5. Add the spring onions (scallions) and cook gently for a few minutes.

6. Break the eggs into a bowl and beat well.

7. Beat the milk, cream and cheese into the eggs.

8. Add the bacon mixture and season to taste with salt and pepper.

9. Roll out the pastry and line a 9-in (23-cm) flan tin (pan).

10. Pour the filling mixture into the pastry case.

11. Bake in a fairly hot oven, 400°F/200°C (Gas Mark 6), for 35 minutes.

<u>CAN BE FROZEN</u>

Cheese Pudding

This is a high energy dish and suitable for those with chewing and swallowing difficulties.

Imperial/metric	Serves 4	American
12 fl oz (340ml)	milk	1½ cups
2 oz (55g)	margarine	¼ cup
3 oz (85g)	stale bread, cubed	1½ cups
3 oz (85g)	Cheddar/New York Cheddar cheese, grated	¾ cup
	salt	
	freshly ground black pepper	
1 tsp	mustard	1 tsp
3	eggs	3

1. Gently heat the milk with the margarine, but do not let it boil. Mix in salt, pepper and mustard.
2. Arrange the bread cubes in an ovenproof dish, sprinkle the cheese over them, then pour the milk mixture over the top.

3. Beat the eggs well and fold into the mixture.
4. Bake at 425°F/220°C (Gas Mark 7) for 30 minutes.

Barbecue Sauce

A tasty addition to chicken, spare ribs, pork chops or beefburgers. It can be added to meat during cooking or served separately. It is suitable for those experiencing taste changes.

Imperial/metric	Serves 4	American
2 oz (55g)	butter	¼ cup
1 tbs	brown sugar	1 tbs
¼ pt (200ml)	ketchup/catsup	⅔ cup
1 tbs	mustard powder	1 tbs
1 tbs	Worcestershire sauce	1 tbs
1	large onion, minced	1
	salt and freshly ground black pepper to taste	
	cayenne pepper to taste	

1. Melt the butter, then add the sugar and, when it is dissolved, add the ketchup (catsup).
2. Mix the mustard powder with the Worcestershire sauce and add to the pan.
3. Add the onion, salt and pepper and simmer for half an hour.

CAN **BE FROZEN**

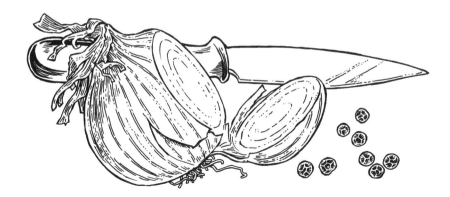

Creamed Spinach

This dish is suitable for those with chewing and swallowing difficulties.

Imperial/metric	*Serves 4*	American
2 lb (900g)	fresh spinach	2 lb
1 oz (30g)	butter	2 tbs
2 tbs	double/heavy cream	2 tbs
	salt	
	freshly ground black pepper	

1. Wash the spinach well and remove the tough stalks, then put it in a saucepan with a couple of tbs of water.
2. Heat the spinach slowly, stirring it occasionally. Leave it on a low heat, cover and cook for 10 minutes or until it is soft.

3. Put it in a liquidizer (blender) with the butter, cream, salt and pepper and blend until smooth.
4. Return the creamed spinach to the pan and re-heat it gently.

Chapter 6

Puddings and Desserts

Fruit Whisk

This dish is suitable for those with chewing and swallowing difficulties and also for taste changes.

Imperial/metric	*Serves 4*	American
1 × 10 oz (298g)	tin/can mandarin oranges, drained, reserving the juice	1 × 10 oz
1	mandarin jelly/jello	1
½ pt (285ml)	boiling water	1⅓ cups
	juice of 1 lemon	
1	egg, separated	1
3 fl oz (90ml)	evaporated milk	⅓ cup

1. Arrange the mandarin segments in the bottom of a bowl.

2. Make up the jelly (jello) with the boiling water, stirring until the cubes have dissolved, then add the reserved juice.

3. Add the lemon juice to the egg yolk in a cup. Stand the cup in a bowl of hot water, stirring occasionally with a fork, until it starts to thicken.

4. Pour the egg white into a large bowl and whisk (beat) until stiff. Continue whisking (beating), adding the milk gradually.

5. Pour the jelly (jello) into the egg white mixture, add the egg yolk and gently fold in until it is all thoroughly mixed together.

6. Pour the jelly (jello) mixture over the arranged fruit and chill until it is set.

Wine Jelly Cream

This is an energy dish and is suitable for those with chewing and swallowing problems and taste changes.

Imperial/metric	Serves 4	American
½ oz (15g)	gelatine powder	1 tbs
3 tbs	sugar	3 tbs
½ pt (285ml)	white wine	1⅓ cups
¾ pt (425ml)	milk	2 cups
2	egg yolks	2
1 tbs	cornflour/cornstarch	1 tbs
½ tsp	vanilla essence/extract	½ tsp
5 fl oz (140ml)	fresh double/heavy cream	⅔ cup

1. Heat the gelatine with 2 tbs of the sugar and ¼ pt (140ml) of the wine in a saucepan over gentle heat until the gelatine dissolves.

2. Mix in the remaining wine and then let the mixture cool a little.

3. Pour equal amounts of the mixture into 4 wine glasses and put in the refrigerator at an angle to chill until set.

4. Heat the milk until it is almost boiling, not letting it boil.

5. Whisk the egg yolks, cornflour (cornstarch), vanilla essence (extract) and remaining sugar together until the mixture turns pale.

6. Pour it into the hot milk, stirring all the time.

7. Strain the mixture to remove any lumps, then gently heat it until it thickens sufficiently to coat the back of a wooden spoon.

8. Let the mixture cool.

9. Whip the cream until it is stiff, then fold it into the cooled custard mixture.

10. Once the wine jelly has set, stand the glasses upright and pour in the custard, filling each glass to the same level.

11. Return the glasses to the refrigerator, upright this time, and chill until set.

Milk Jelly

This dish is suitable for those with chewing and swallowing difficulties. For those experiencing taste changes, use a sharp flavour such as lemon or lime.

Imperial/metric	Serves 4	American
1 packet	fruit-flavoured jelly/jello	1 packet
¼ pt (140ml)	boiling water	⅔ cup
¼ pt (140ml)	cold water	⅔ cup
1 × 6 fl oz (170ml)	tin/can evaporated milk, chilled	1 × 6 fl oz

1. Dissolve the jelly (jello) in the boiling water, then mix in the cold water.
2. Whisk (beat) the evaporated milk until it is thick, then combine it with the cold jelly (jello).
3. Pour the mixture into 1 or 4 individual moulds and chill until set.

Lemon Sweet

This is a high energy dish. It is suitable for those with chewing and swallowing difficulties and taste changes.

Imperial/metric	Serves 4	American
1 × 14 oz (397g)	tin/can condensed milk	1 × 14 oz
1 small carton	single/light cream	1 small carton
	Rind and juice of 2 lemons	
	Crystallized lemon or orange slices (optional)	

1. Liquidize (blend) all the ingredients together.
2. Pour the mixture into 4 individual serving dishes and chill for 3 hours.
3. Decorate, if you like, with crystallized lemon or orange slices before serving.

Crème Guineve

This is a high energy dish and is suitable for those with chewing and swallowing difficulties.

Imperial/metric	*Serves 2*	American
2 oz (55g)	plain/unsweetened chocolate, broken into pieces	½ cup
2 tbs	water	2 tbs
2	small/medium eggs, separated	2
	dash of brandy or rum	

1. Melt the chocolate in a bowl over hot water, stirring from time to time.
2. While it is still hot, add the egg yolks.
3. Beat the egg whites until they are stiff, then fold them into the chocolate mixture when it has cooled slightly but is still fluid.

4. Add the brandy or rum.
5. Pour the crème into 2 serving dishes and chill until it is firm.

CAN BE FROZEN

Baked Egg Custard

This dish is suitable for those with chewing or swallowing difficulties.

Imperial/metric	*Serves 4*	American
2	eggs	2
1-2 tbs	sugar	1-2 tbs
½ pt (285ml)	milk	1⅓ cups
1 tsp	grated nutmeg or ground cinnamon	1 tsp

1. Whisk (beat) the eggs and sugar together, then add the milk and mix well.

2. Lightly grease a 1½ pt (850ml/quart) oven-proof dish and strain the egg and milk mixture through a sieve (strainer) into the dish. This removes any parts of the egg white which do not mix well.

3. Sprinkle the top with the nutmeg or cinnamon and place the dish in a baking tin half-filled with hot water.

4. Bake at 325°F/170°C (Gas Mark 3) for 45 minutes.

Chocolate Mousse

This is a high energy dish and is suitable for those with chewing and swallowing difficulties.

Imperial/metric	Serves 4	American
½ pt (285ml)	single/light cream	1⅓ cups
6 oz (170g)	plain/unsweetened chocolate	1½ cups
1	medium/large egg	1
½ tsp	vanilla essence/extract	½ tsp

1. Heat the cream in a saucepan until it is just below boiling point — do not let it boil.

2. Pour it into a liquidizer (blender).

3. Break up the chocolate into the liquidizer (blender) and blend.

4. Add the egg and vanilla essence (extract) and blend.

5. Pour the mousse into 4 ramekin dishes and put in the refrigerator to chill until it has set.

Malvern Pudding

This is a high energy dish and is suitable for those with chewing and swallowing difficulties.

Imperial/metric	Serves 4	American
2½ oz (70g)	butter	5 tbs
1 lb (455g)	cooking/tart apples, peeled and sliced	1 lb
2 oz (55g)	sugar	4 tbs
1 oz (30g)	plain/all-purpose flour	¼ cup
¾ pt (425ml)	milk	2 cups
1	egg, beaten	1
1 oz (30g)	demerara/raw brown sugar	2 tbs

1. Put 1 oz (30g/2 tbs) of the butter in a saucepan and melt.

2. Add the apples and 1 oz (30g/2 tbs) of the sugar and cook gently, stirring, until the mixture is soft and thick.

3. Remove the pan from the heat and pour the mixture into a lightly greased ovenproof dish.

4. Melt 1 oz (30g/2tbs) of the butter in a saucepan and stir in the flour.

5. Cook gently for a couple of minutes without browning the flour.

6. Remove the pan from the heat and gradually add the milk, stirring well as you do so.

7. Return the pan to the heat and bring to the boil, stirring all the time, and then let it simmer for 2 minutes.

8. Remove the pan from the heat once more and stir in 1 oz (30g/2 tbs) of the sugar.

9. Add the beaten egg a little at a time and stir well.

10. Return the pan to the heat and cook for about 1 minute, stirring, then pour the sauce over the apple mixture in the dish.

11. Dot the top with the remaining butter and sprinkle with the demerara (raw brown) sugar.

12. Put the dish under a hot grill (broiler) and cook until the sugar has caramelized.

Apple Snow

This dish is suitable for those with chewing and swallowing difficulties and taste changes.

Imperial/metric	*Serves 4*	American
2 lb (900g)	cooking/tart apples, peeled and chopped	3 cups
	grated rind of 1 orange	
	juice of 1 orange	
3 tbs	honey	3 tbs
2	egg whites	2

1. Put the apple, orange rind, orange juice and honey in a saucepan and cook gently until soft, then mash to a pulp.

2. Beat the egg whites until they are stiff, then fold them into the apple purée.

3. Pour the snow into 4 bowls or glasses and chill until firm.

Crème Caramel

This dish is suitable for those with chewing and swallowing difficulties.

Imperial/metric	*Serves 4*	American
3 oz (85g)	sugar	½ cup
3	eggs	3
3 tbs	sugar	3 tbs
23 fl oz (645 ml)	milk	3 cups
1 tsp	vanilla essence/extract	1 tsp

1. Melt the sugar gently in a heavy-bottomed saucepan until it is pale brown.

2. Beat together the eggs and sugar, then gradually add the milk and vanilla, mixing it all together very well.

3. Pour the caramel into a heavy ovenproof dish, then pour the custard mixture on top.

4. Place the dish in a pan of hot water and bake at 300°F/150°C (Gas Mark 2) for 40 minutes or until the custard has set.

Lemon Pudding

This is a high energy dish and is suitable for those with chewing and swallowing difficulties.

Imperial/metric	Serves 6	American
1 heaped tbs	cornflour/cornstarch	1 heaped tbs
¾ pt (425ml)	cold water	2 cups
5 oz (140g)	sugar	1 cup
	rind and juice of 2 lemons	
2	eggs, beaten	2
2 × 7-in (18-cm)	sponge cakes/round layers of pound cake	2 × 7 in

1. Mix the cornflour (cornstarch) carefully with the cold water.

2. Add the sugar, lemon rind and juice and the eggs.

3. Pour the mixture into a saucepan and, on a gentle heat, stir it continually until it thickens and has a consistency like custard. Keep it from boiling.

4. Layer the mixture and the sponge cake in a glass bowl, alternating them, and finish with the mixture.

5. Chill until set and serve with fresh double cream for a real treat.

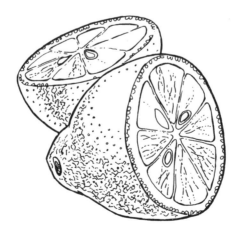

Apple Sponge Pudding

This dish is suitable for those with chewing and swallowing difficulties and is also high in energy.

Imperial/metric	Serves 4	American
1 lb	Bramley/tart apples, peeled and sliced	1 lb
1 oz (25g)	sugar	2 tbs
2 tbs	cold water	2 tbs
1 tsp	ground cinnamon	1 tsp
	Sponge Topping	
4 oz (115g)	margarine	½ cup
4 oz (115g)	caster/superfine sugar	⅔ cup
2	eggs	2
4 oz (115g)	self-raising/self-rising flour	1 cup
1 tbs	warm water	1 tbs
1 tbs	flaked/slivered almonds (optional)	1 tbs

1. Put the apples, sugar and water into a saucepan, bring to the boil and then simmer very gently until the apples are soft, but not pulpy.

2. Pour the cooked apples into a lightly greased 2½ pt (1.4l/1¼ quart) ovenproof dish, sprinkle the cinnamon over the apples and leave to cool slightly. The cooked apple can be frozen at this point, though it should be thawed thoroughly before adding the sponge topping.

3. Meanwhile, prepare the sponge topping. Beat the margarine and sugar until the mixture is soft and pale.

4. Beat in the eggs and stir in the flour and warm water.

5. Spread the sponge mixture over the cooked apple and sprinkle with the flaked (slivered) almonds if using.

6. Bake for 30 minutes at 350°F/180°C (Gas Mark 4) or until it is golden. Serve with ice-cream, cream, yoghurt or custard.

CAN BE FROZEN

Sunshine Pudding

This dish is high in energy. Simply omit the sultanas (golden seedless raisins) if you have chewing and swallowing difficulties.

Imperial/metric	*Serves 2*	American
3 oz (85g)	fresh white breadcrumbs	1½ cups
2 oz (55g)	sultanas/golden seedless raisins	⅓ cup
	grated rind of 1 lemon	
½ pt (285ml)	milk	1½ cups
2 oz (55g)	sugar	½ cup
1	egg	1
	grated nutmeg	

1. Lightly grease a 1-pt (570ml/½ quart), shallow ovenproof dish.

2. In a bowl, mix together the breadcrumbs, sultanas (golden seedless raisins) and lemon rind.

3. Gently heat the milk and sugar together until just warm.

4. Lightly beat the egg and add it to the warmed milk.

5. Pour the milk mixture over the breadcrumb mixture, stir it all together, then pour it into the prepared dish.

6. Sprinkle the grated nutmeg over the top and bake for 30 minutes at 375°F/190°C (Gas Mark 5) until set in the centre.

Home-made Cream

This is a high energy recipe.

Imperial/metric	Serves 4	American
4 oz (115g)	unsalted butter	1 stick
¼ pt (140ml)	milk	⅔ cup
1 tsp	gelatine powder	1 tsp
1-2 tsp	caster/superfine sugar	1-2 tsp
1-2 drops	vanilla essence/extract	1-2 drops

1. Cut the butter into pieces and place in a pan with the milk.

2. Sprinkle the gelatine over this mixture and heat gently, but do not let it boil.

3. Stir until all the gelatine has melted.

4. Stir in the sugar and vanilla essence (extract).

5. Pour the cream into a liquidizer (blender) and mix on high speed for 30 seconds, then pour it into a bowl.

6. Cover the bowl and chill the cream for at least 3 hours, but preferably overnight.

7. Whip before serving if desired.

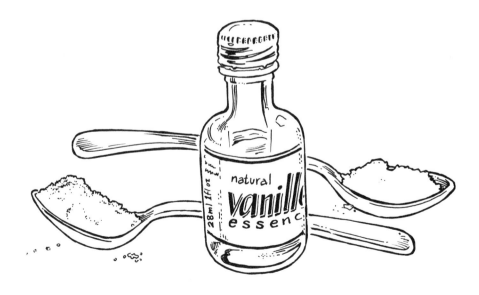

Lemon Delight

This dish is suitable for those with chewing and swallowing difficulties and taste changes.

Imperial/metric	*Serves 4*	American
4 oz (115g)	margarine	½ cup
3 oz	caster/superfine sugar	⅓ cup
	juice and rind of 2 lemons	
3	eggs, separated	3
3 oz (85g)	self-raising/self-rising flour	½ cup
9 fl oz (255ml)	milk	1¼ cups

1. Beat together the margarine, sugar and lemon rind.

2. Stir in the egg yolks, flour, lemon juice and milk, making sure that you combine all the ingredients well.

3. Beat the egg whites until they are stiff, then fold them into the mixture.

4. Pour the mixture into a greased pie dish.

5. Bake at 350°F/180°C (Gas Mark 4) for 40 minutes, or until centre feels set when pressed lightly.

Gentle Pudding

This is a high energy dish and is suitable for those with chewing and swallowing difficulties.

Imperial/metric	*Serves 4*	American
3	eggs, separated	3
2 tbs	sugar	2 tbs
1 tsp	vanilla sugar	1 tsp
3 tbs	double/heavy cream	3 tbs
1 tbs	plain/all-purpose flour	1 tbs
	rind of 1 orange, grated	

1. Butter and lightly flour a deep gratin or soufflé dish.
2. Whisk (beat) the egg yolks, sugar and vanilla sugar until the mixture is very thick and creamy.
3. Blend the cream into the egg yolk mixture.
4. Whisk (beat) the egg whites until they are very stiff.
5. Fold the egg whites, spoonful by spoonful, alternately with the flour, into the egg yolk mixture.
6. Sprinkle in the orange rind.
7. Pour the mixture into the prepared dish and bake in a fairly hot oven, 400°F/200°C (Gas Mark 6) for about 15 minutes, until it has lightly browned on top.
8. Serve at once.

Raspberry Mêlée

This is a high energy dish and is suitable for those with chewing and swallowing difficulties and taste changes.

Imperial/metric	Serves 6	American
1	egg white, stiffly beaten	1
3 oz (85g)	icing/confectioner's sugar	½ cup
½ pt (285ml)	cream, whipped	1⅓ cups
4 oz (115g)	raspberries, fresh or frozen	1 cup
	few drops vanilla essence/extract	

1. Fold the egg white and sugar into the cream, then spoon a third of it into a separate bowl.
2. Mash the raspberries with a fork and stir the purée into the reserved third of the cream mixture.
3. Flavour the remainder of the cream mixture with the vanilla essence (extract).
4. Take 6 individual dishes and layer the raspberry cream mixture with the vanilla cream.
5. Chill until firm.

Banana Whip

This is a high energy dish and is suitable for those with chewing and swallowing difficulties.

Imperial/metric	Serves 4	American
4	bananas	4
1	egg white	1
1 oz (30g)	caster/superfine sugar	2 tbs
¼ pt (140ml)	double/heavy cream	⅔ cup

1. Mash the bananas to form a smooth purée.
2. Whisk (beat) the egg white until it is stiff, then fold in the sugar.

3. Fold the banana purée and the egg white gently into the cream.
4. Spoon the mixture into 4 individual dishes and chill until firm.

Creamy Fruit Topping

This is a delicious topping which is ideal for cooked, tinned or fresh fruit of any kind. This is a high energy dish and is suitable for those with chewing and swallowing difficulties.

Imperial/metric	Serves 4	American
6 oz (170g)	curd/ricotta cheese	¾ cup
1 tbs (15g)	caster/superfine sugar	1 tbs
¼ pt (140ml)	double/heavy cream	⅔ cup

1. Mix the cheese with the sugar, then beat in the cream.

2. Pour the mixture into a serving dish and chill until firm.

Lemon and Pineapple Soufflé

This is a high energy dish and is suitable for those with chewing and swallowing difficulties and taste changes.

Imperial/metric	Serves 4	American
3	eggs, separated	3
½ tsp	lemon rind, grated	½ tsp
4 oz (115g)	caster/superfine sugar	⅔ cup
¼ oz (1 packet/envelope)	gelatine	1 packet
¼ pt (140ml)	pineapple juice, warmed	⅔ cup
2 tbs	lemon juice	2 tbs
8 oz (225g)	tinned/canned pineapple, chopped	1⅔ cups
¼ pt (140ml)	double/heavy cream	⅔ cup

1. Put the egg yolks, lemon rind and sugar in a bowl and whisk (beat) until it is of a creamy consistency.

2. Soak the gelatine in the warmed pineapple juice until the granules have dissolved, then add the lemon juice and let cool.

3. Add the gelatine mixture and the pineapple to the egg mixture.

4. Whisk (beat) the cream until it is thick, then fold it into the egg, gelatine and pineapple mixture.

5. Whisk (beat) the egg whites until they are stiff and fold this, too, into the mixture.

6. Pour the mixture into a soufflé dish or large bowl and refrigerate until it is cold and set.

Chapter 7

Cakes

Cherry and Almond Cake

This dish is high in energy and is suitable as a nourishing snack.

Imperial/metric	*Makes 15 portions*	American
6 oz (170g)	margarine	¾ cup
6 oz (170g)	caster/superfine sugar	1 cup
3	eggs	3
4 oz (115g)	self-raising/self-rising flour	1 cup
4 oz (115g)	ground almonds	2 cups
3 oz (85g)	glacé/candied cherries, washed and halved	½ cup

1. Beat the margarine and sugar together until the mixture becomes soft and pale.
2. Beat in the eggs one at a time.
3. Stir in the sifted flour and almonds and the cherries.
4. Pour the mixture into a greased 11-in (28-cm) × 7-in (18-cm) cake tin (pan) and bake at 350°F/180°C (Gas Mark 4) for 40-45 minutes, or until the cake springs back when pressed lightly.
5. Leave the cake in the tin (pan) to cool, then cut it into 15 squares.

CAN BE FROZEN

72

Guinness Cake

This is a high energy recipe.

Imperial/metric	Makes 12-16 portions	American
8 oz (225g)	butter or margarine	1 cup
8 oz (225g)	soft brown sugar	1¼ cups
2	eggs, beaten	2
12 oz (340g)	raisins	2 cups
12 oz (340g)	plain/all-purpose flour	3 cups
3 tsp	baking powder	3 tsp
1 tsp	mixed spice	1 tsp
¼ pt (140ml)	Guinness	⅔ cup

1. Beat the butter or margarine with the sugar until the mixture becomes fluffy and pale.

2. Add the beaten eggs, a little at a time, combining well after each addition.

3. Stir in the raisins.

4. Gradually fold in the flour, baking powder and mixed spice.

5. Mix in the Guinness until the batter is smooth.

6. Pour it into an 8-in (20-cm) round cake tin (pan) and bake in a cool or slow oven 300°F/150°C (Gas Mark 2) for 2-2½ hours until cake is firm and springs back when pressed lightly.

7. Leave in the tin to cool. Then turn out. Wrap the cake in foil or greaseproof (waxed) paper and keep for 2 days before eating.

Lemon Cake

This is a high energy recipe and is suitable for those with chewing and swallowing difficulties and for taste changes.

Imperial/metric	*Makes 8-10 slices*	American
4 oz (115g)	soft margarine	½ cup
4 oz (115g)	caster/superfine sugar	⅔ cup
2	eggs	2
4 oz (115g)	self-raising/self-rising flour	1 cup
¼ tsp	baking powder	¼ tsp
1 tbs	lemon curd	1 tbs
1 tbs	lemon juice	1 tbs
	Icing/frosting	
2 oz (55g)	soft margarine	¼ cup
4 oz (155g)	icing/confectioner's sugar	⅔ cup
1 dsp	lemon juice	2 tsp

1. Put the margarine, caster (superfine) sugar, eggs, flour, baking powder, lemon curd and lemon juice in a mixing bowl and beat until all the ingredients are well mixed (this should take approximately 3-4 minutes).
2. Pour the mixture into a round, greased 7½-in (29-cm) cake tin (pan) and bake at 350°F/180°C (Gas Mark 4) for 40-45 minutes until cake springs back when pressed lightly. Leave to cool in the tin for 10 minutes, then remove and place on a wire rack.
3. Beat the margarine, icing (confectioner's) sugar and lemon juice together until the mixture is soft, then spread it over the top of the cake.

CAN BE FROZEN

Virginia's Orange Cake

This dish is high in energy and is suitable for those with chewing and swallowing difficulties and taste changes.

Imperial/metric	*Makes 12-16 slices*	American
8 oz (225g)	margarine	1 cup
8 oz (225g)	caster/superfine sugar	1⅓ cup
3	eggs	3
1 tsp	vanilla essence/extract	1 tsp
8 oz (225g)	plain/all-purpose flour	2 cups
1 tsp	baking powder	1 tsp
	Topping	
	grated rind and juice of 1 orange	
	grated rind and juice of 1 lemon	
8 oz (225g)	brown sugar	1⅓ cup

1. Beat the margarine and sugar together until the mixture becomes soft and pale.

2. Beat in the eggs, one at a time.

3. Fold in the sifted flour and baking powder.

4. Pour the mixture into a well-greased ring tin (tube pan) and bake at 350°F/180°C (Gas Mark 4) for 45 minutes or until the cake springs back when lightly pressed. Leave in the tin for 10 minutes and then place on a wire rack.

5. Meanwhile, put the orange and lemon rind, juice and sugar in a saucepan and bring to the boil, then let it cool and pour it over the cake while the cake is still hot.

CAN BE FROZEN

Melting Moments

This is a high energy recipe.

Imperial/metric		American
3 oz (85g)	margarine	⅓ cup
1 oz (30g)	white lard or solid vegetable fat/shortening	2 tbs
3 oz (85g)	caster/superfine sugar	½ cup
½	egg	½
1 tsp	vanilla essence/extract	1 tsp
5 oz (140g)	self-raising/self-rising flour	1¼ cups
	desiccated/shredded coconut	
2 oz (55g)	glacé/candied cherries, halved	½ cup

1. Beat the fat and sugar together until the mixture becomes soft and pale.

2. Beat in the egg and the vanilla essence (extract).

3. Stir in the flour and mix well.

4. With wet hands, roll the mixture into small balls and then roll them in the coconut.

5. Place them on a greased baking sheet and press lightly with the back of a fork (they will spread so leave plenty of space between them).

6. Bake at 350°F/180°C (Gas Mark 4) for 15 minutes, then decorate with cherries.

Microwave Lemon Curd

This is a high energy recipe.

Imperial/metric		American
8 oz (225g)	caster/superfine sugar	1¼ cups
4 oz (115g)	unsalted butter	1 stick
	grated rind of 1 lemon	
	juice of 3 lemons	
4	eggs, beaten well	4

1. Put the sugar, butter, lemon rind and juice in a microwave bowl.

2. Cook on high for 8 minutes, stirring frequently (during this time the sugar should dissolve and the mixture come to a rolling boil).

3. Cook on high for a further minute or two.

4. Add the eggs.

5. Put back in the microwave, cook on high and stir every minute until the mixture thickens.

6. Pot it while the mixture is still warm.

7. Once cool, store the curd in the refrigerator.

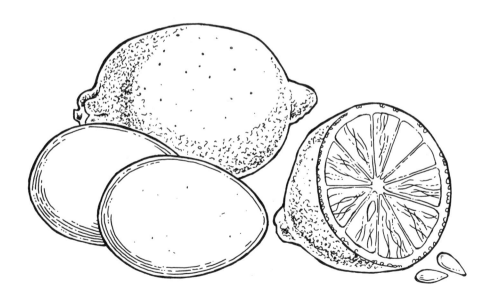

Chapter 8

Nourishing Drinks

Fortified Milk

Use in place of ordinary milk in cooking for soups, milk puddings, nourishing drinks and so on. This is a high protein milk.

Imperial/metric	*Makes 1 pt (570ml/2½ cups)*	American
1 pt (570ml)	full cream milk	2½ cups
2 oz (55g)	dried skimmed milk powder	⅔ cup

1. Put the milk and milk powder in a liquidizer (blender) and blend for 15 seconds until well mixed. Keep in the refrigerator until needed.

Mocha Shake

This is a high energy, high protein nourishing drink.

Imperial/metric	*Serves 1*	American
7 fl oz (200ml)	vanilla liquid nutritional supplement	¾ cup
2 tsp	instant coffee	2 tsp
1 tbs	chocolate milk shake syrup	1 tbs
1 scoop	ice-cream	1 scoop
½ tsp	cinnamon	½ tsp
3 tsp	glucose polymer powder	3 tsp

1. Liquidize (blend) all the ingredients and serve immediately.

Yoghurt Cooler

This is a high energy, high protein nourishing drink.

Imperial/metric	*Serves 1*	American
5 fl oz (140ml)	milk	⅔ cup
3 fl oz (90ml)	fruit yoghurt	⅓ cup
3 tsp	glucose polymer powder	3 tsp

1. Blend all the ingredients and serve immediately.

Fizzy Fruit Cup

This is a high energy nourishing drink.

Imperial/metric	*Serves 1*	American
3 fl oz (90ml)	fruit-flavoured high energy glucose drink	⅓ cup
3 fl oz (90ml)	lemonade	⅓ cup

1. Chill the ingredients.

2. Mix the ingredients together and serve immediately.

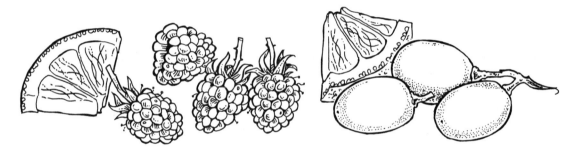

Sunrise Special

This is a high energy nourishing drink.

Imperial/metric	*Serves 1*	American
3 fl oz (90ml)	apricot high energy glucose drink	⅓ cup
3 fl oz (90ml)	orange juice	⅓ cup

1. Chill the ingredients.

2. Mix the ingredients together and serve immediately.

Somerset Surprise

This is a high energy nourishing drink.

Imperial/metric	*Serves 1*	American
3 fl oz (90ml)	apple-flavoured high energy glucose drink	⅓ cup
2 fl oz (60ml)	apple juice	¼ cup
2 fl oz (60ml)	lemonade	¼ cup

1. Chill the ingredients.

2. Mix the ingredients together and serve immediately.

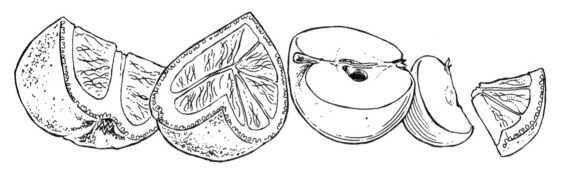

Fruit Juice Special

This is a high energy nourishing drink.

Imperial/metric	*Serves 1*	American
7 fl oz (200ml)	fruit juice	¾ cup
4 tsp	glucose polymer powder	4 tsp

1. Mix both the ingredients together and serve.

Apple Fizz

This is a high energy nourishing drink.

Imperial/metric	Serves 1	American
3 fl oz (90 ml)	apple-flavoured high energy glucose drink	⅓ cup
3 fl oz (90ml)	ginger ale	⅓ cup

1. Chill the ingredients.

2. Mix the ingredients together and serve immediately.

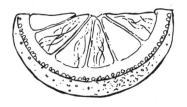

Citrus Cup

This is a high energy nourishing drink.

Imperial/metric	Serves 1	American
3 fl oz (90ml)	lemon-flavoured high energy glucose drink	⅓ cup
3 fl oz (90ml)	orange juice	⅓ cup

1. Chill the ingredients.

2. Mix the ingredients together and serve immediately.

Coffee Calypso

This is a high energy, high protein nourishing drink.

Imperial/metric	*Serves 1*	American
1 serving	powdered vanilla nutritional supplement	1 serving
½ pt (285ml)	milk	1⅓ cups
1 tsp	instant coffee	1 tsp
1 scoop	ice-cream	1 scoop
4 tsp	glucose polymer powder	4 tsp

1. Liquidize (blend) all the ingredients together.   **2.** Pour into a tall glass and serve with a straw.

Fruit Connection

This is a high energy, high protein nourishing drink.

Imperial/metric	*Serves 1*	American
4 oz (115g)	tinned/canned fruit, e.g., apricots, peaches	1 cup
½ serving	powdered vanilla nutritional supplement	½ serving
5 fl oz (140ml)	milk	⅔ cup
1 tsp	sugar (optional)	1 tsp
3 tsp	glucose polymer powder	3 tsp

1. Liquidize (blend) the fruit.
2. Add the powdered nutritional supplement, milk, sugar, if using, and the glucose polymer powder and liquidize (blend) all the ingredients together.
3. Pour into a glass and serve.

After Eight

This is a high energy, high protein nourishing drink.

Imperial/metric	*Serves 1*	American
½ serving	powdered chocolate nutritional supplement	½ serving
5 fl oz (140ml)	milk	⅓ cup
	few drops peppermint essence/extract	
3 tsp	glucose polymer powder	3 tsp

1. Liquidize (blend) all the ingredients together.　　**2.** Serve immediately.

Tarzan's Treat

This is a high energy, high protein nourishing drink.

Imperial/metric	*Serves 1*	American
½ serving	powdered vanilla nutritional supplement	½ serving
5 fl oz (140ml)	milk	⅓ cup
½	ripe banana	½
	or	
1-2 tsp	banana milkshake flavouring	1-2 tsp
3 tsp	glucose polymer powder	3 tsp

1. Liquidize (blend) all the ingredients together.　　**2.** Serve immediately.

Tangy Ice-cream

This dish is high in energy and suitable for those with chewing and swallowing difficulties.

Imperial/metric	*Serves 1*	American
5 oz (140g)	caster/superfine sugar	⅔ cup plus 2 tbs
5 fl oz (140ml)	milk, warmed	⅔ cup
5 fl oz (140ml)	double/heavy cream	⅔ cup
	juice of 2 lemons	

1. Dissolve the sugar in the milk then leave to cool.

2. Whip the cream until it is thicker but not forming peaks.

3. Beat it into the sugared milk.

4. Stir in the lemon juice, then freeze.

5. After 2 hours, remove from the freezer and whip until smooth, then refreeze.

Sparkly Fruit Cup

This is a high energy nourishing drink.

Imperial/metric	*Serves 1*	American
5 fl oz (140ml)	blackcurrant high energy glucose drink	⅔ cup
2 fl oz (60ml)	apple juice	¼ cup
2 fl oz (60ml)	soda water	¼ cup

1. Chill the ingredients.

2. Mix them together and serve immediately.

Fruit Float

This is a high energy, high protein nourishing drink.

Imperial/metric	*Serves 1*	American
7 fl oz (200ml)	fruit-flavoured liquid nutritional supplement, e.g. peach, strawberry, chilled	¾ cup
3 fl oz (90ml)	soda water	⅓ cup
1 scoop	vanilla ice-cream	1 scoop

1. Mix the liquid nutritional supplement with the soda water in a tall glass.

2. Float the ice-cream on the top and then serve immediately with a straw.

Desert Island Delight

This is a high energy nourishing drink.

Imperial/metric	*Serves 1*	American
5 fl oz (140ml)	milk	⅔ cup
1 fl oz (30ml)	pineapple juice	2 tbs
1 scoop	vanilla ice-cream	1 scoop
4 tsp	glucose polymer powder	4 tsp

1. Liquidize (blend) all the ingredients together.

2. Serve in a tall glass with a cocktail umbrella.

Fruit Smoothie

This recipe is suitable for those with chewing and swallowing difficulties and taste changes.

Imperial/metric	*Serves 1*	American
10 oz (285g)	soft fruit (any combination)	2 cups
4 fl oz (120ml)	natural/plain yoghurt	½ cup
4 fl oz (120ml)	milk	½ cup
	honey, sugar or cream to taste (optional)	

1. Chop the fruit and put it into a liquidizer (blender).

2. Add the yoghurt and milk and liquidize (blend) for approximately 1 minute until smooth.

	Dessert variation	
2 tbs	gelatine powder*	2 tbs
4 fl oz (120ml)	hot water	½ cup

1. Dissolve the gelatine in the water.
2. As steps 1 and 2 above but add the gelatine mixture before liquidizing (blending).

3. Pour the mixture into a bowl and chill in the refrigerator for 1-2 hours until it has set.

* If using fresh pineapple use three times the normal amount of gelatine.

Part 3

Recipes for Healthy Eating

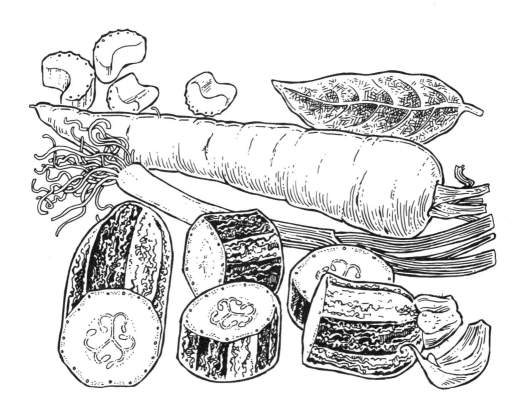

Chapter 9

Breakfasts

Swiss Breakfast Apple Muesli

This dish is high in fibre and low in fat.

Imperial/metric	Serves 2	American
2	dessert/sweet apples, cored and diced	2
	juice of ½ lemon	
1 oz (30g)	(English) walnuts	3 tbs
¼ pt	semi-skimmed/low-fat milk	⅔ cup
4 tbs	rolled oats	4 tbs
2 oz (55g)	seedless raisins or sultanas/golden seedless raisins	⅓ cup
1 serving	fresh fruit, e.g., banana, strawberries	1 serving

1. Put the apple, lemon juice, walnuts and milk in a liquidizer (blender) and blend for 20 seconds.
2. Pour the mixture into a bowl, stir in the rolled oats and raisins or sultanas (golden seedless raisins) and leave overnight.
3. Serve with the fresh fruit.

Banana Muffins

This recipe is high in fibre.

Imperial/metric	Makes 18 small muffins	American
3	large ripe bananas	3
4 oz (115g)	brown sugar	¾ cup
1	egg	1
6 oz (170g)	plain/all-purpose flour	1½ cups
¾ tsp	salt	¾ tsp
1 tsp	bicarbonate of soda/baking soda	1 tsp
1 tsp	baking powder	1 tsp

1. Pre-heat the oven to a moderate 350°F/180°C (Gas Mark 4) and grease a bun (muffin) tin (pan), or 2 or more if you have them. You can also use paper cases if you like.
2. In a large bowl, beat together the bananas, sugar and egg until smooth.
3. Sift together the flour, salt, bicarbonate of soda (baking soda) and baking powder.

4. Fold it gradually into the banana mixture and mix gently until well combined.
5. Spoon the muffin batter into the greased bun (muffin) tins (pans) or paper cases to two-thirds capacity to allow the mixture to rise.
6. Bake for 15 minutes or until golden brown and repeat step 5 until all the batter has been used.

CAN BE FROZEN

Apple Muffins

This recipe is high in fibre and relatively low in fat and sugar.

Imperial/metric	Makes 12 large muffins	American
4 oz (115g)	self-raising/self-rising wholemeal/wholewheat flour	1 cup
4 oz (115g)	self-raising/self-rising white flour	1 cup
1 tsp	cinnamon	1 tsp
2 oz (55g)	brown sugar	⅓ cup
2	eggs	2
2 oz (55g)	margarine	¼ cup
6 fl oz (179ml)	milk	⅔ cup + 2 tbs
2	apples, peeled and grated	2

1. Grease a bun (muffin) tin (pan), or more if you have them. Use paper cases for the muffins if you like. Pre-heat the oven to 375°F/190°C (Gas Mark 5).

2. Sift together the flours and cinnamon, then add the sugar.

3. Add the eggs, margarine and milk and mix well until you have a smooth batter.

4. Fold in the apples. Spoon into greased muffin tins.

5. Bake for 20-25 minutes.

<u>**CAN BE FROZEN**</u>

Breakfast Banana Nog

This recipe is low in fat and moderately high in fibre.

Imperial/metric	Serves 1	American
7 fl oz (200ml)	semi-skimmed/low-fat milk	¾ cup
3 fl oz	low-fat plain yoghurt	⅓ cup
1	ripe banana	1
1 tsp	honey	1 tsp

1. Place the milk, yoghurt, banana and honey in a liquidizer (blender) and blend until smooth.

2. Serve immediately or use as an accompaniment to muesli.

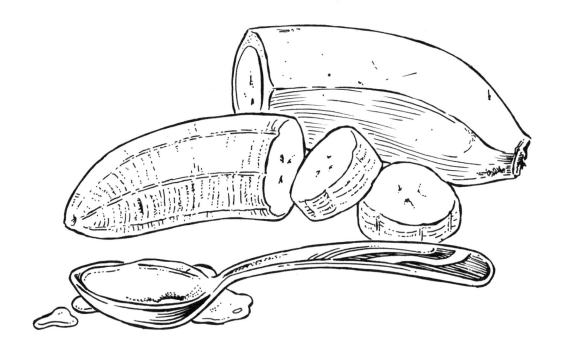

Chapter 10

Starters

Orange and Carrot Soup

This dish is low in fat.

Imperial/metric	Serves 4	American
1	onion, chopped	1
1 oz (30g)	margarine	2 tbs
1 lb (455g)	carrots, diced	1 lb
1⅔ pt (1l)	chicken stock	3¾ cups
1 carton	frozen orange juice concentrate, thawed	1 carton
⅙ pt (100ml)	natural/plain yoghurt	½ cup
	grated rind of 1 orange	

1. Soften the onion in the margarine.
2. Add the carrots and stir together.
3. Add the chicken stock and simmer until the carrots are tender.
4. Pour the mixture into a liquidizer (blender) and blend until it is the texture you like.

5. Add the orange juice a little at a time to taste.
6. Pour the soup back into the pan, reheat, stir in the yoghurt, then serve immediately
7. Garnish with the orange rind.

CAN BE FROZEN
(before orange juice and yoghurt are added)

Tomato and Bean Soup

This dish is low in fat.

Imperial/metric	*Serves 4*	American
1	medium onion, finely chopped	1
1 tbs	corn oil	1 tbs
3 oz (85g)	lean ham or bacon, chopped	1-2 slices
1 × 4 oz (115g)	tin/can tomato purée/paste	1 × 4 oz
2 pt (1.1l)	water	5 cups
	pinch of mixed herbs	
1	bay leaf	1
2	cabbage leaves, finely chopped	2
1 oz (30g)	soup pasta	¼ cup
1 × 5 oz (140g)	tin/can baked beans	1 × 5 oz
	Parmesan cheese, grated to garnish (optional)	

1. Fry the onion in the corn oil and add the ham or bacon.

2. Add the tomato purée (paste), water and herbs.

3. Simmer for at least an hour.

4. Ten minutes before serving, add the cabbage leaves, pasta and baked beans. Simmer for the remaining 10 minutes.

5. Remove the bay leaf before serving and serve with the Parmesan cheese sprinkled in the centre of the bowl.

CAN BE FROZEN

Lentil Soup

This dish is high in fibre and low in fat.

Imperial/metric	Serves 4	American
1 tbs	sunflower oil	1 tbs
1	medium onion, finely chopped	1
1 clove	garlic, crushed/minced	1 clove
2	medium carrots, chopped	2
1 pt (570ml)	vegetable stock	2½ cups
½ tsp	dried mixed herbs	½ tsp
	or	
1 tsp	fresh herbs, finely chopped	1 tsp
	pinch chilli powder	
½ tsp	turmeric powder	½ tsp
4 oz (115g)	red lentils	½ cup
2 tbs	tomato purée/paste	2 tbs
	salt	
	freshly ground black pepper	

1. Heat the oil in a saucepan and sauté the onion and garlic for 5 minutes.
2. Add the carrot and cook for a further 5 minutes.
3. Add the vegetable stock, herbs, chilli powder, turmeric, lentils, tomato purée (paste) and salt and pepper.
4. Simmer for 45 minutes and adjust the seasoning if necessary.
5. Serve with wholemeal bread.

CAN BE FROZEN

Chapter 11

Main Courses

Kidneys in Cider

This dish is low in fat.

Imperial/metric	*Serves 4*	American
	lamb kidneys (3 per person)	
	cider	
	chicken stock/bouillon cube	
¼ lb (115g)	mushrooms, sliced	1½ cups
	freshly ground black pepper	

1. Slice the kidneys, and remove the central core, wash them and put them in a casserole dish.
2. Pour enough cider over the kidneys to just cover them and crumble in the chicken stock (bouillon) cube and add the mushrooms and pepper.
3. Cover and cook in the centre of a moderate oven, 350°F/180°C (Gas Mark 4), for about 2½ hours.

CAN BE FROZEN

Low-fat Beefburgers

This dish is low in fat.

Imperial/metric	Serves 4	American
1 lb (455g)	lean braising steak/beef chuck or	1 lb
	lean shoulder steak, minced/ground	
1	small onion, chopped	1
1 tsp	Worcestershire sauce	1 tsp
½ tsp	mustard	½ tsp
2 tsp	parsley, finely chopped	2 tsp
2 tsp	tomato purée/paste	2 tsp
	salt	
	freshly ground black pepper	
3 oz (75g)	fresh wholemeal/wholewheat breadcrumbs	1½ cups
1	egg	1
	vegetable oil	

1. Mix the beef, onion, Worcestershire sauce, mustard, parsley, tomato purée (paste), salt, pepper and breadcrumbs together well.

2. Add the egg and mix thoroughly.

3. Turn the mixture out onto a floured surface and, using floured hands, divide the mixture into 8 equal pieces and shape into ½-in (1-cm) thick flat rounds. (Freeze at this point if desired.)

4. Brush lightly with vegetable oil.

5. Place under a hot grill (broiler) and cook for 8 minutes on each side.

6. Serve in a wholemeal (wholewheat) roll with a side salad.

CAN BE FROZEN

Beef Oriental

This dish is moderately low in fat.

Imperial/metric	Serves 4	American
1¼ lb (565g)	steak, cubed	1¼ lb
1	onion, chopped	1
1	sweet/green pepper, chopped	1
1 tbs	cooking oil	1 tbs
4 oz (115g)	mushrooms, sliced	2 cups
1 clove	garlic, crushed/minced	1 clove
½ pt (285ml)	stock	1⅓ cups
3 tbs	vinegar	3tbs
2 tbs	sherry	2 tbs
½ tsp	soy sauce	½ tsp
½ oz (15g)	sugar	1 tbs
1-2 tbs	cornflour/cornstarch	1-2 tbs

1. Fry the steak, onion and pepper briefly in the oil, just enough to seal the meat, and transfer to a casserole dish.

2. Add the mushrooms and garlic.

3. Mix the stock, vinegar, sherry, soy sauce and sugar in a saucepan over a medium heat until the sugar has dissolved.

4. Pour the sauce into the casserole and mix with the meat and vegetables.

5. Cook in a moderate oven, 350°F/180°C (Gas Mark 4), for at least 1½ hours.

6. Mix the cornflour (cornstarch) to a cream with a little water, add it to the casserole and cook for a further half hour.

CAN BE FROZEN

Pork and Apple Casserole

This dish is low in fat.

Imperial/metric	Serves 4	American
4	large, lean pork chops	4
1 tsp	dried sage	1 tsp
1	onion, sliced	1
	salt and pepper	
¼ pt (140ml)	dry/hard cider	⅔ cup
1	cooking/tart apple, cored and sliced	1
2	tomatoes, sliced	2

1. Put the chops down the centre of a shallow casserole dish and sprinkle the sage over them.
2. Put the onion slices down each side of the chops.
3. Season and pour the cider over the onions.
4. Cover tightly with foil and cook in a moderate oven, 350°F/180°C (Gas Mark 4), for 1 hour.

5. Place the apple and tomato slices over the onions and return the casserole to the oven until the apple is tender (approximately 10-15 minutes).
6. Adjust the seasoning if necessary, then remove the foil and let the meat brown a little before serving.

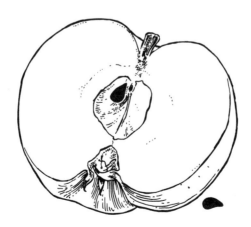

Veal à la Med

This dish is low in fat and high in fibre.

Imperial/metric	Serves 4	American
1 tbs	cooking oil	1 tbs
1	large onion, sliced	1
2 cloves	garlic, crushed/minced	2 cloves
1 lb (455g)	lean stewing veal, cubed	1 lb
	salt	
	freshly ground black pepper	
1 tsp	dried thyme	1 tsp
1 tsp	dried oregano	1 tsp
1 tbs	tomato purée/paste	1 tbs
¾ pt (425ml)	chicken stock	2 cups
1 × 14 oz (395g)	tin/can tomatoes	1 × 14 oz
8 oz (225g)	aubergine/eggplant or courgette/zucchini, cut into chunks	1½ cups
1	large sweet/green pepper, sliced	1
4 oz (115g)	button mushrooms	2 cups
6 oz (170g)	wholemeal/wholewheat pasta shells	1½ cups
1 tsp	fresh basil, chopped, to garnish	1 tsp

1. Heat the oil in a large casserole dish, then add the onion and garlic.
2. Cover and cook for 2 minutes until soft.
3. Add the veal and cook, stirring, until it is lightly browned.
4. Add the remaining ingredients except the pasta and basil.
5. Cover and cook in a moderate oven, 350°F/180°C (Gas Mark 4), for 45 minutes.
6. Stir in the pasta shells, cover and cook for 20 minutes more or until the pasta is tender.
7. Check the seasoning and serve, garnishing each dish with the basil.

CAN BE FROZEN
(Cool and freeze after stage 5. To use, thaw, add the pasta and then follow steps 6 and 7.)

Spicy Chicken Casserole

This dish is low in fat.

Imperial/metric	*Serves 4*	American
1	onion, peeled	1
1 blade	mace	1 blade
6	peppercorns	6
1 sprig	thyme	1 sprig
	rind of 1 lemon	
	few sprigs of parsley	
1 tsp	salt	1 tsp
	freshly ground black pepper	
1½ pt (850ml)	water	3¾ cups
1	chicken	1
	or	
4	chicken breasts	4
	or	
6	chicken thighs, skinned	6
2 tbs	cornflour/cornstarch	2 tbs
1 pt (570ml)	chicken stock	2½ cups
2 tsp	curry powder	2 tsp
2 tbs	redcurrant jelly	2 tbs
5 fl oz (140ml)	low-fat natural/plain yoghurt	⅔ cup

1. Put the onion in the saucepan with the mace, peppercorns, thyme, lemon rind, parsley, salt and pepper and add the water and chicken pieces and cover.

2. Bring to the boil, then simmer for 1-1¼ hours.

3. Remove the chicken, then strain and reserve the cooking liquor, skimming off the fat when it has cooled.

4. Cut the chicken meat into cubes or strips.

5. Mix the cornflour (cornstarch) to a paste with some of the cooled stock. Warm the remainder of the stock until it is nearly at boiling point then pour it onto the paste and mix.

6. Return the stock to the pan, add the curry powder and redcurrant jelly, bring to the boil, stirring continuously, and cook for 2 minutes until thick. Then, add the chicken and heat through. (Freeze now if desired.)

7. Add the yoghurt just before serving and adjust the seasoning if necessary. Reheat but do not let the casserole boil.

CAN BE FROZEN

Chicken Stir Fry

This dish is low in fat.

Imperial/metric	Serves 4	American
4	chicken breasts, skinned	4
2 tbs	cornflour/cornstarch	2 tbs
2 tbs	soy sauce	2 tbs
3 tbs	white wine	3 tbs
2 tbs	sunflower oil	2 tbs
1	small onion, peeled and sliced	1
2	sweet/green peppers, deseeded and sliced	2
2 cloves	garlic, crushed/minced	2 cloves
3 tbs	blanched almonds	3 tbs
	salt	
	freshly ground black pepper	

1. Cut the chicken into thin strips and toss in the cornflour (cornstarch). Add the soy sauce and wine to the chicken and coat well.

2. Heat 1 tbs of the oil. Fry the onion, pepper, garlic and almonds for 5 minutes. Remove from the pan and keep warm.

3. Heat the remaining oil, drain the chicken and fry for 5 minutes.

4. Return the onion, pepper and almonds to the pan. Heat through for 5-10 minutes, stirring all the time.

5. Stir in the remaining soy sauce and wine, salt and pepper.

6. Serve with brown rice or wholemeal noodles.

Chicken Kebabs

This dish is low in fat.

Imperial/metric	*Serves 4*	American
2	chicken breasts, skinned	2
½	sweet/green pepper	½
½	sweet/red pepper	½
12	button mushrooms	12
8	cherry tomatoes	8
8	pickling onions, skinned	8
2	bananas, sliced	2
1 tbs	sunflower oil	1 tbs
1 tsp	soy sauce	1 tsp
	freshly ground black pepper	

1. Cut the chicken and pepper into 1-in (3-cm) cubes and squares.

2. Thread the chicken, pepper, mushrooms, tomatoes, onions and bananas onto 4 skewers, distributing the ingredients evenly.

3. Mix the oil, soy sauce and black pepper together and brush it over the kebabs.

4. Place the kebabs under a pre-heated grill (broiler) and cook for 10-12 minutes, turning them frequently and brush them with the oil mixture again if they seem to be getting a little dry.

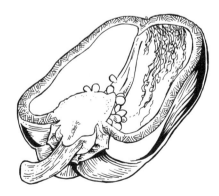

Chicken Tikka

This dish is low in fat.

Imperial/metric	*Serves 2-3*	American
1½ lb (680g)	boned chicken	1½ lb
	juice of 1 lemon	
	pinch of salt	
½	fresh green chilli, chopped	½
2 tsp	garam masala	2 tsp
½ in (2.5cm)	fresh root ginger, chopped	½ in
1 clove	garlic, crushed/minced	1 clove
½	onion, chopped	½
10 fl oz (285ml)	natural/plain yoghurt	1⅓ cups
	lemon wedges to serve	

1. Cut the chicken into cubes, marinate them in the lemon juice and salt for 20 minutes.
2. Combine all the other ingredients and blend in a liquidizer (blender) or food processor to form a paste.
3. Strain the paste over the chicken and lemon juice and stir well.

4. Marinate for a further 6-24 hours.
5. Pre-heat the grill (broiler) to very hot, thread the chicken onto skewers and grill (broil) the chicken for 10 minutes.
6. Serve with the lemon wedges.

Grilled (Broiled) Spring Chicken

This dish is low in fat.

Imperial/metric	Serves 4	American
2 cloves	garlic, crushed/minced	2 cloves
	juice of 1½ lemons	
1 tsp	cayenne pepper	1 tsp
	freshly ground black pepper	
2 tbs	olive oil	2 tbs
4	chicken breast portions, skinned	4
1-2 tbs	Dijon mustard	1-2 tbs
2 oz (55g)	fresh breadcrumbs	1 cup

1. Combine the garlic, lemon, cayenne pepper, black pepper and oil.
2. Marinade the chicken pieces in this mixture for an hour or so.
3. Pre-heat the grill (broiler) to moderately high and grill (broil) the chicken portions for 10 minutes each side.
4. Turn again, brush with the mustard, sprinkle with breadcrumbs and grill (broil) until the crumbs are golden.

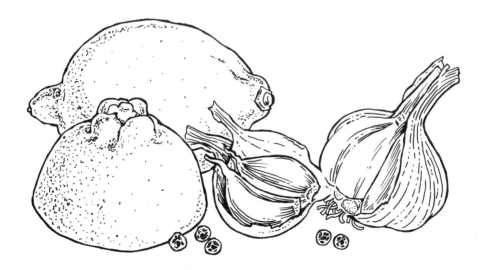

Chicken and Apricots

This dish is low in fat.

Imperial/metric	*Serves 4*	American
1 × 1 lb (455g)	tin/can apricots	1 × 1 lb
4	chicken pieces	4
4 tbs	plain/all-purpose flour	4 tbs
2 tbs	cooking oil	2 tbs
1	onion, chopped	1
6 tbs	chicken stock	6 tbs

1. Drain the apricots, reserving the juice, and slice them.

2. Coat the chicken with flour and brown in the oil in a frying pan (skillet).

3. Remove the chicken to a small casserole dish.

4. Cook the onion in the frying pan (skillet) until it begins to brown.

5. Add the remaining flour, apricots and juice and the chicken stock and bring to the boil, stirring.

6. When it has thickened pour it over the chicken.

7. Cover and cook in a warm oven, 325°F/170°C (Gas Mark 3), for 1¼ hours.

CAN BE FROZEN

Chicken Hawaii Style

This dish is low in fat.

Imperial/metric	Serves 4	American
2 oz (55g)	plain/all-purpose flour	½ cup
1 tsp	paprika	1 tsp
	pinch of salt and pepper	
1	chicken, jointed	1
2 tbs	cooking oil	2 tbs
1 × 9 oz (255g)	tin/can crushed pineapple	1 × 9 oz
	grated rind of 1 orange	
¼ pt (140ml)	orange juice	⅔ cup

1. Season the flour with the paprika, salt and pepper.

2. Coat the chicken joints in the flour and brown on both sides in the oil, which needs to be hot.

3. Put the chicken in a casserole dish.

4. Season them with salt and pepper and add the pineapple and its juice, the orange rind and orange juice.

5. Cover and cook in a moderate oven, 375°/190°C (Gas Mark 5), for 1 hour, removing the lid for the last 15 minutes.

CAN BE FROZEN

Slimline Turkey

This dish is low in fat.

Imperial/metric	Serves 4	American
4	turkey breast fillets	4
	salt and pepper to taste	
1	onion, sliced	1
1	bay leaf	1
4 oz (115g)	button mushrooms	2 cups
¼ pt (140ml)	chicken stock	⅔ cup
½	cucumber, sliced	½
	fresh parsley, chopped, to garnish	

1. Season the turkey with salt and pepper, then brown in a non-stick pan without any fat, sautéing it over a medium heat for a few minutes.
2. Add the onion, bay leaf, mushrooms and chicken stock.
3. Cover and bring to the boil, then simmer for 20 minutes.

4. Add the sliced cucumber, check the seasoning and adjust if necessary and simmer for a few minutes.
5. Discard the bay leaf, lift out the turkey fillets first, spoon some sauce over each one and then garnish with the parsley.

CAN BE FROZEN

Turkey Fillet with Grapes

This dish is low in fat.

Imperial/metric	*Serves 4*	American
1 lb (455g)	turkey breasts, skinned and boned	1 lb
1 tbs	cooking oil	1 tbs
2	spring onions/scallions, cut into 2-in lengths	2
	freshly ground black pepper	
2 tbs	dry sherry	2 tbs
2 tbs	water	2 tbs
1½ tbs	soy sauce	1½ tbs
8 oz (225g)	green grapes, halved and seeded	2 cups

1. Cut the turkey into thin strips and brown them quickly in the oil.

2. Add the spring onions (scallions) and cook for a further 2 minutes.

3. Add all the remaining ingredients, except for 2 oz (55g/½ cup) of the grapes.

4. Stir, cover and simmer gently for 5 minutes.

5. Serve garnished with the remaining grapes.

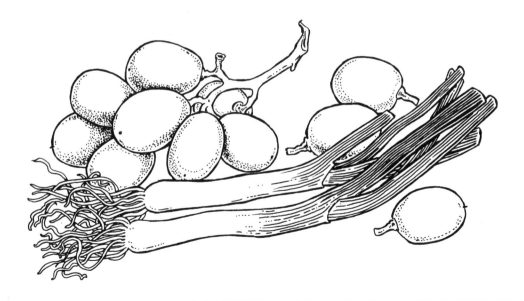

Fish Risotto

This dish is high in fibre and low in fat.

Imperial/metric	Serves 4	American
	juice of 1 lemon	
1½ lb (680g)	white fish fillets	1½ lb
2 tbs	sunflower oil	2 tbs
8 oz (225g)	brown rice	1 cup
2 cloves	garlic, crushed/minced	2 cloves
7 fl oz (200ml)	vegetable stock	⅓ cup
7 fl oz (200ml)	white wine	⅓ cup
	salt and freshly ground black pepper to taste	
1 lb (455g)	tomatoes	2⅔ cups
1 bunch	parsley	1 bunch
2 tbs	Cheddar/New York Cheddar cheese, grated	2 tbs

1. Pour the lemon juice over the fish, leave it to marinate for 10 minutes, then cut it into cubes.
2. Heat the oil in a large, heavy pan and braise the rice on medium heat, stirring occasionally.
3. Add the garlic and stir.
4. Place the cut fish onto the rice and then add the stock, wine, salt and pepper.
5. Cover the pan and simmer for 20 minutes.

6. Meanwhile, skin the tomatoes and chop the parsley.
7. Add the tomatoes to the risotto and cook for a further 5 minutes or until the liquid has been absorbed.
8. Add the parsley and cheese and then serve immediately with a salad.

Oven-baked Rainbow Trout

This dish is low in fat.

Imperial/metric	Serves 2	American
2	rainbow trout, gutted and left whole	2
	juice of ½ lemon	
2 tbs	white wine	2 tbs
1 tbs	fresh parsley, finely chopped	1 tbs
	salt	
	freshly ground black pepper	
	slices of lemon to garnish	

1. Pre-heat the oven to 350°F/180°C (Gas Mark 4).

2. Wash the trout and dry with kitchen paper towel.

3. Put the fish in a dish lined with a piece of foil large enough to wrap loosely around the fish.

4. Pour the lemon juice and wine over the trout, sprinkle the parsley over and season with salt and pepper.

5. Pull the foil round the fish and pleat together, leaving each end slightly open and curled up from the dish.

6. Bake in the oven for 40 minutes. Serve with slices of lemon.

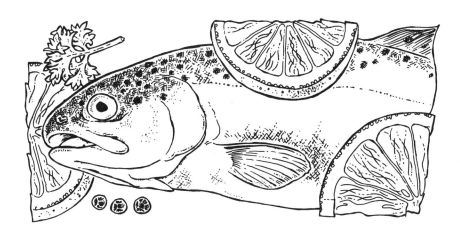

Paella

This dish is low in fat and high in fibre.

Imperial/metric	Serves 4	American
8 oz (225g)	brown rice	1 cup
1	chicken stock/bouillon cube	1
1¼ pt (710ml)	water	3 cups
½ tsp	turmeric	½ tsp
½ tbs	sunflower oil	½ tbs
2 rashers	bacon, fat trimmed and finely chopped	2 rashers
1	large onion, peeled and chopped	1
1	sweet/green pepper, seeded and chopped	1
2 oz (55g)	mushrooms, chopped	¾ cup
¾ lb (340g)	prawns/shrimp	¾ lb
	freshly ground black pepper	

1. Put the rice, chicken stock (bouillon) cube, water and turmeric in a large saucepan.

2. Bring to the boil and simmer, covered, for 25 minutes or until the rice is cooked and all the water has been absorbed.

3. Heat the oil in a frying pan (skillet) and stir-fry the bacon, onion and pepper for 5 minutes.

4. Add the cooked rice, mushrooms, prawns and black pepper and heat through, stirring occasionally.

CAN BE FROZEN

Fish and Rice Bake

This dish is high in fibre and low in fat.

Imperial/metric	Serves 4	American
1 lb (455g)	white fish	1 lb
8 oz (225g)	brown rice	1 cup
1 pt (570ml)	water	2½ cups
2 oz (55g)	low-fat spread	¼ cup
½ pt (285ml)	chicken stock, hot	1⅓ cups
4 oz (115g)	onion, chopped	⅔ cup
6 oz (170g)	celery, chopped	1 cup
4 oz (115g)	peas	⅔ cup
2½ oz (70g)	fresh breadcrumbs	1¼ cups
2	eggs, beaten	2

1. Boil or poach the fish, drain and flake.

2. Put the rice in the water in a pan and simmer covered, for approximately 25 minutes until tender.

3. Melt the low-fat spread in the chicken stock.

4. Combine all ingredients in a casserole dish, cover and bake in a moderate oven, 350°F/180°C (Gas Mark 4), for 30 minutes.

5. Remove the cover and bake for a further 15 minutes.

Plaice with Red Peppers

This dish is low in fat.

Imperial/metric	*Serves 4*	American
8	plaice fillets	8
2	sweet/red peppers	2
2 tbs	soy sauce	2 tbs
	juice of 1 lemon	
1 tsp	ground ginger	1 tsp
8 × 10-in (25-cm)	square pieces of foil	8 × 10-in
	oil for greasing	
	Sauce	
4 tbs	soy sauce	4 tbs
2 tsp	tomato purée/paste	2 tsp
2 tbs	sunflower oil	2 tbs

1. Cut the plaice fillets in half lengthways.

2. Cut each pepper into 8 pieces.

3. Mix the soy sauce and lemon juice together.

4. Brush the plaice with some of this mixture and reserve the rest.

5. Sprinkle the plaice with the ground ginger.

6. Put a piece of pepper on the end of each plaice strip and roll it up so that the pepper ends up in the middle.

7. Oil each piece of foil and put 2 plaice rolls on each one.

8. Bring the edges of the foil together, fold and seal.

9. Put the parcels in a steamer.

10. Lower the steamer into a large pan of boiling water and steam for about 15 minutes. Put the plates nearby to warm.

11. Meanwhile, mix the remaining soy sauce and lemon juice mix with the sauce ingredients, pour into a saucepan and bring the sauce to simmering point, but do not let it boil.

12. Unwrap each parcel of fish and put the rolls on the warmed plates. Serve the sauce separately.

Cod Provençale

This dish is low in fat.

Imperial/metric	Serves 4	American
	Marinade	
¼ pt (140ml)	dry white wine	⅔ cup
2 tbs	lemon juice	2 tbs
1 tsp	dried basil	1 tsp
1 tsp	black pepper	1 tsp
4	cod steaks	4
1	large onion, chopped	1
1 clove	garlic, crushed/minced	1 clove
1 × 14 oz (395g)	tin/can tomatoes	1 × 14 oz
1 tbs	olive oil	1 tbs

1. Combine the marinade ingredients and marinade the fish for 2-3 hours.
2. Fry the onion, garlic and tomatoes in the oil.
3. Remove the fish from the marinade and add the marinade to the pan.

4. Bring the mixture to the boil, then reduce the heat to low and simmer until the sauce thickens.
5. Add the cod steaks and cook for about 10 minutes. The fish is done when it flakes easily.

CAN BE FROZEN

Nut-stuffed Peppers

This dish is vegetarian and high in fibre.

Imperial/metric	Serves 4	American
4	sweet/green peppers	4
8 oz (225g)	ground mixed nuts	2 cups
4 oz (115g)	wholemeal/wholewheat breadcrumbs	2 cups
1	onion, peeled and chopped	1
1 clove	garlic, crushed/minced	1 clove
2 tbs	tomato purée/paste	2 tbs
2 tsp	dried mixed herbs	2 tsp
	or	
1 tbs	fresh mixed herbs, chopped	1 tbs
	salt	
	freshly ground black pepper	
1 × 14 oz (395g)	tin/can tomatoes, drained (juice reserved), and chopped	1 × 14 oz
2	eggs, beaten	2

1. Slice off the top of the peppers and de-seed, then blanch them in boiling water for 5 minutes and drain well.
2. Mix the nuts, breadcrumbs, onion, garlic, tomato purée (paste), herbs, salt and pepper. Add the tomatoes and eggs and mix well.

3. Arrange the peppers in an ovenproof dish and fill each with the nut mixture. Pour the reserved tomato juice into the dish around the peppers.
4. Bake at 375°F/190°C (Gas Mark 5) for 1-1¼ hours. (Cover with foil if the peppers start to brown.) Serve immediately.

CAN BE FROZEN

Vegetable and Cashew Risotto

This dish is vegetarian, high in fibre and relatively low in fat.

Imperial/metric	Serves 4	American
8 oz (225g)	brown rice	1 cup
	pinch of salt	
1 tbs	sunflower oil	1 tbs
1	onion, finely chopped	1
1 clove	garlic, crushed/minced	1 clove
1	sweet/red pepper, seeded and chopped	1
1	sweet/green pepper, seeded and chopped	1
1	stick/stalk celery, chopped	1
8 oz (225g)	mushrooms, sliced	2 cups
3 oz (75g)	sweetcorn kernels	½ cup
4 oz (115g)	cashew nuts	¾ cup
	salt and freshly ground black pepper	

1. Put the rice in a saucepan, cover with water, add the salt, bring to the boil and simmer for 25-30 minutes until cooked. Then, rinse in boiling water and drain well.

2. While the rice is cooking, heat the oil in a large pan, add the onion and garlic and cook over a medium heat for 5 minutes, stirring occasionally.

3. Add the peppers, celery, mushrooms, sweetcorn, cashew nuts, season to taste with salt and pepper and cook over the same medium heat for 5 minutes, stirring occasionally. Cover and cook over a low heat for an additional 5-10 minutes.

4. Add the cooked rice, stir everything together and continue to heat for 3 minutes until all ingredients are heated through, then serve immediately.

Vegetable Groundnut Stew

This dish is vegetarian and high in fibre.

Imperial/metric	Serves 4	American
1 tbs	sunflower oil	1 tbs
1	large onion, peeled and sliced	1
1 clove	garlic, crushed/minced	1 clove
1	sweet/red pepper, deseeded and sliced	1
8 oz (225g)	carrots, peeled and sliced	½ lb
6 oz (170g)	button mushrooms	3 cups
8 oz (225g)	tomatoes, skinned and chopped	½ lb
1 pt (570ml)	vegetable stock	2½ cups
2 tsp	paprika	2 tsp
1-in (2.5cm)	root ginger, grated	1-in
4 oz (115g)	crunchy peanut butter	1 cup
	salt	
	freshly ground black pepper	
4 oz (115g)	frozen peas	⅔ cup

1. Heat the oil in a saucepan. Fry the onions, garlic and pepper for 5 minutes, stirring occasionally.

2. Add the carrots, mushrooms, tomatoes, vegetable stock, paprika, root ginger, peanut butter, salt and pepper and bring to the boil. Cook for 15-20 minutes.

3. Add the peas and cook for a further 10 minutes.

4. Serve with brown rice and a green salad.

Mushroom and Chestnut Wholewheat/Wholemeal Lasagne

This is a vegetarian dish that is high in fibre and relatively low in fat.

Imperial/metric	*Serves 4*	American
4 oz (115g)	dried chestnuts	¾ cup
1 tbs	sunflower oil	1 tbs
1	onion, chopped	1
2 cloves	garlic, crushed/minced	2 cloves
12 oz (340g)	mushrooms, sliced	4½ cups
1 × 14 oz (375g)	tin/can tomatoes	1 × 14 oz
2 tbs	tomato purée/paste	2 tbs
2 tsp	fresh herbs, chopped	2 tsp
1 tsp	or dried herbs	1 tsp
4 tbs	red wine	4 tbs
	salt	
	freshly ground black pepper	
1½ tbs	cornflour/cornstarch	1½ tbs
¾ pt (425ml)	semi-skimmed/low-fat milk	2 cups
6 oz (170g)	no-cook wholemeal/wholewheat lasagne	6 oz
4 oz (115g)	strong Cheddar/New York Cheddar cheese, grated	1 cup

1. Place the chestnuts in a large pan and cover with water. Bring to the boil and simmer on a low heat for 35-40 minutes, or until the chestnuts are tender.
2. Heat the oil in a large pan, and fry the onion and garlic until soft, stirring occasionally.
3. Add the mushrooms and sauté on medium heat for 3 minutes.
4. Add the tomatoes, tomato purée (paste), herbs, wine, salt and pepper, bring to the boil and simmer for 15 minutes. Add the drained chestnuts. (Freeze the sauce at this point if desired.)
5. To make the white sauce, mix the cornflour (cornstarch) with enough of the milk to make a smooth paste.

6. Warm the remainder of the milk in a pan until just below boiling. Pour it onto the cornflour (cornstarch) mixture, return it to the pan, bring it to the boil slowly, stirring constantly until it has thickened.
7. Grease an ovenproof dish approximately 8 × 10 in (20 × 25cm) and place a layer of the lasagne in the bottom. Cover with half the mushroom and chestnut sauce, then a layer of pasta, then the rest of the sauce and finish with a layer of pasta.
8. Pour the white sauce over the top layer of the pasta and sprinkle the cheese over the top.
9. Bake at 375°F/190°C (Gas Mark 5) for 45 minutes.

CAN BE FROZEN

Vegetarian Moussaka

This dish is vegetarian and high in fibre.

Imperial/metric	Serves 4	American
1¼ lb (565g)	aubergines/eggplants	1¼ lb
	salt	
4 tbs	sunflower oil	4 tbs
1	onion, chopped	1
12 oz (340g)	mushrooms, sliced	4½ cups
1 × 14 oz (395g)	tin/can chopped tomatoes	1 × 14 oz
¼ tsp	ground cinnamon	¼ tsp
1 tbs	fresh oregano, chopped	1 tbs
	salt and freshly ground black pepper	
1½ tbs	cornflour/cornstarch	1½ tbs
¾ pt (425ml)	semi-skimmed/low-fat milk	2 cups
1	egg, separated	1
4 oz (115g)	Parmesan cheese, grated	1 cup

1. Slice the aubergines (eggplants) and layer in a colander or sieve, sprinkling each layer with salt. Weigh down with a plate and leave for 20 minutes, then rinse well and pat dry with kitchen paper towel.
2. Heat the oil in a large frying pan (skillet) and fry half the aubergines (eggplants) for 5 minutes on each side. Remove them from the pan (skillet) and repeat for the rest of the slices and remove them from the pan also.
3. Add the onion to the pan and cook for 5 minutes, then add the mushrooms and cook for 5 minutes.
4. Add the tomatoes, cinnamon and oregano, bring to boil and simmer uncovered for 15 minutes, then season to taste with salt and pepper. (Freeze at this point if desired.)
5. Put the cornflour (cornstarch) in a jug, add a small amount of the milk and mix to a smooth paste.

Warm the remainder of the milk until it is nearly boiling.
6. Pour the hot milk onto the cornflour (cornstarch) paste, stirring, and return the mixture to the pan. Bring it to the boil, stirring constantly, until the sauce has thickened, then remove it from the heat. Stir in the egg yolk and half of the cheese, and season with salt and pepper. Make sure it is all well mixed.
7. Whisk the egg white in a large bowl until it is stiff, then fold it gently into the cheese sauce.
8. Put half the aubergine (eggplant) slices in a 2 pt (1.1l/quart) ovenproof dish. Cover with half the mushroom and tomato mixture, then half the cheese sauce. Repeat these three layers, finishing with the cheese sauce. Sprinkle the remaining Parmesan on the top.
9. Bake at 350°F/180°C (Gas Mark 4) for 45 minutes until the cheese is golden brown.

CAN BE FROZEN

Scone Pizza

This recipe is high in fibre.

Imperial/metric	*Serves 4*	American
1	large, onion, chopped	1
½	sweet/green pepper, chopped	½
2 oz (55g)	mushrooms, sliced	¾ cup
1 × 14 oz (395g)	tin/can tomatoes, drained	1 × 14 oz
1 dsp	dried mixed herbs	2 tsp
	salt	
	freshly ground black pepper	
1 tbs	tomato purée/paste	1 tbs
6 oz (170g)	wholemeal/wholewheat self-raising/self-rising flour	1½ cups
2½ oz (70g)	margarine	¼ cup plus 1 tbs
3 fl oz (90ml)	milk	⅓ cup
6 oz (170g)	Cheddar/New York Cheddar cheese, grated	1½ cups

1. Put the onion, pepper, mushrooms, tomatoes, herbs, salt, pepper and tomato purée (paste) in a pan and bring to the boil. Cover and simmer for 15 minutes, then let it cool slightly.
2. Put the flour in a mixing bowl and rub the margarine into it until it resembles breadcrumbs.
3. Add the milk and mix to a soft dough, then, on a floured board, roll it out to a 9-10-in (25-28-cm) round and put it on a greased baking sheet.

4. Strain any excess liquid from the tomato mixture, then spread it over the scone base to within 1 in (2.5cm) from the edge.
5. Sprinkle the cheese over the top.
6. Bake the pizza at 400°F/200°C (Gas Mark 6) for 20-25 minutes or until the cheese is bubbling and golden brown.

CAN BE FROZEN

Jacket Potatoes

This dish is low in fat and makes a delicious nourishing snack.

Imperial/metric	Serves 4	American
4	large potatoes, washed	4
1 oz (30g)	bacon, chopped	1 slice
1 tsp	onion, chopped	1 tsp
1 tsp	fresh parsley, chopped	1 tsp
1 oz (30g)	low-fat spread	1 tbs
1	egg, beaten	1

1. Bake the potatoes in a hot oven until cooked.
2. Cut each one in half and scoop out the potato from the skins.
3. Mix this with all the other ingredients except the egg and then put the mixture back into the shells.

4. Brush the tops with the egg.
5. Bake in a hot oven, 425°F/220°C (Gas Mark 7), for 10-15 minutes.

Mushrooms à la Grecque

This dish is vegetarian and low in fat.

Imperial/metric	Serves 4	American
4	carrots, finely diced	4
1 lb (455g)	onions, finely chopped	1 lb
1 tbs	olive oil	1 tbs
8 oz (225g)	mushrooms, sliced	½ lb
¼ pt (140ml)	wine vinegar	⅔ cup
8	tomatoes, skinned	8
1 tbs	tomato purée/paste	1 tbs
	bouquet garni	
	salt and freshly ground black pepper, to taste	
	fresh parsley, chopped, to garnish	

1. Fry the carrots and onion in the olive oil until they are golden brown.
2. Add the mushrooms and stir for 1 minute.
3. Add the vinegar and the rest of the ingredients, except the parsley.

4. Simmer gently for 15 minutes.
5. Remove the bouquet garni, leave to cool, then chill well.
6. Sprinkle with the parsley and serve with fresh bread.

Dry Potato Curry

This dish is vegetarian and low in fat.

Imperial/metric	Serves 4	American
1	medium onion, chopped	1
1½ tbs	cooking oil	1½ tbs
¼ tsp	fenugreek	¼ tsp
¼ tsp	fennel seeds	¼ tsp
½ tsp	black mustard seeds	½ tsp
1 tsp	turmeric powder	1 tsp
½ tsp	chilli powder	½ tsp
2 tbs	fresh coriander/cilantro leaves, chopped	2 tbs
1 tsp	salt	1 tsp
1 lb (455g)	potatoes, cubed	1 lb
2 fl oz (60ml)	hot water	¼ cup
1 tsp	garam masala	1 tsp
1 tbs	lemon juice	1 tbs

1. Cut the potatoes into cubes.
2. Fry the onion gently in oil for 5 minutes.
3. Add the fenugreek, fennel and mustard seeds.
4. When the mustard seeds begin to pop, add the turmeric, chilli powder, coriander (cilantro) and salt.

5. Add the potato and the hot water and stir together well.
6. Cover with a tight-fitting lid and simmer gently on a very low heat for 20 minutes.
7. Sprinkle the garam masala and lemon juice in and cook for another 10 minutes.

CAN BE FROZEN

125

Curried Okra

This dish is vegetarian and low in fat.

Imperial/metric	Serves 4	American
2 tsp	ground cumin	2 tsp
2 tsp	ground coriander/cilantro	2 tsp
½ tsp	turmeric	½ tsp
	salt to taste	
	chilli powder to taste	
½ tbs	cooking oil	½ tbs
½ lb (225g)	okra, big and even-sized	½ lb
¼ tsp	mustard seeds	¼ tsp
¼ tsp	cumin seeds	¼ tsp
3-4	tomatoes, chopped	3-4

1. Mix the cumin, coriander (cilantro) and turmeric and salt and chilli to taste with a little of the oil.

2. Top and tail the okra and wipe clean instead of rinsing them.

3. Make a 1-in (2.5-cm) long slit down the okra without going right through and stuff with ⅓ tsp of the spicy paste.

4. Heat the oil in a pan and, when it is hot, add the mustard and cumin seeds. Heat them until they pop.

6. Add the tomatoes and cook for 1 minute.

7. Add the okra, cover with a tight-fitting lid and cook over a very low heat until the okra are soft.

<u>**CAN BE FROZEN**</u>

Stuffed Aubergines (Eggplant)

This dish is vegetarian, high in fibre and low in fat.

Imperial/metric	Serves 4	American
4	large aubergines/eggplants	4
2 oz (55g)	peeled cooked prawns/shrimp	¾ cup
1	small onion, chopped	1
2	medium tomatoes, chopped	2
1 clove	garlic, crushed/minced	1 clove
	pinch dried basil	
	pinch dried oregano	
2 oz (55g)	fresh, fine, wholemeal/wholewheat breadcrumbs	1 cup

1. Boil the aubergines (eggplants) in lots of water for a few minutes until the skins start to wrinkle.

2. Cut each into half along its length and scoop out the flesh from the skins.

3. Mix the flesh with the prawns, onion, tomato, garlic, basil and oregano and spoon it back into the skins.

4. Bake in a moderate oven, 350°F/180°C (Gas Mark 4), for about 30 minutes.

5. Sprinkle the breadcrumbs over the stuffed aubergines (eggplants) and brown under a hot grill (broiler).

CAN BE FROZEN

Rice and Beans

This dish is vegetarian and high in fibre.

Imperial/metric	Serves 4	American
6 oz (170g)	dried kidney beans	1 cup
1 clove	garlic, peeled	1 clove
4 oz (115g)	solid coconut cream	½ cup
	black pepper to taste	
	pinch thyme	
8 oz (225g)	brown rice	2 cups

1. Rinse the beans, soak them in plenty of water overnight and then drain them.
2. Put the beans in a pressure cooker with water up to 1 in (2.5cm) above the level of the beans.
3. Pressure cook for 20 minutes.
4. Lift the cover, add the other ingredients, except the rice, and simmer gently for 20 minutes.
5. Add the rice, bring to the boil, stir and reduce the heat to simmering point.
6. Cover and simmer for approximately 20 minutes until all the liquid has been absorbed.

CAN BE FROZEN

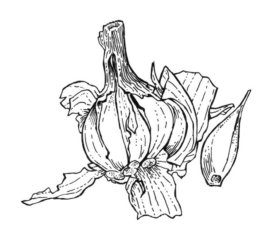

Spanish Rice

This dish is low in fat and may be served hot or cold.

Imperial/metric	Serves 4	American
1 tbs	olive oil	1 tbs
1	large onion, chopped	1
1	sweet/green pepper, diced	1
2	sweet/red peppers, diced	2
1 × 14 oz (395g)	tin/can tomatoes, chopped	1 × 14 oz
2 oz (55g)	green olives, stoned/pitted	½ cup
10 oz (285g)	button mushrooms, sliced	3¾ cups
1 tsp	dried oregano	1 tsp
½ tsp	dried basil	½ tsp
1 tsp	black pepper	1 tsp
6 oz (170g)	rice, cooked, preferably brown	1 cup

1. Heat the oil in a large pan and fry the onions until they are soft.

2. Add the peppers and stir-fry for 5 minutes.

3. Add the tomatoes and their juice, the olives, mushrooms, herbs and pepper and simmer for 3-4 minutes.

4. Add the rice and simmer for a further 3-4 minutes until the rice is heated through.

CAN BE FROZEN

Chick Peas with Coconut

This dish is high in fibre.

Imperial/metric	Serves 4	American
1	medium onion, chopped	1
½ tbs	cooking oil	½ tbs
1 tsp	powdered nutmeg	1 tsp
2 tsp	cardamom seeds, crushed	2 tsp
4 fl oz (120ml)	white wine	½ cup
	pinch of pepper	
2 oz (55g)	coconut cream	¼ cup
1 × 15 oz (425g)	tin/can chick peas/garbanzos	1 × 15 oz

1. Fry the onion lightly in the oil until softened (approximately 5 minutes).
2. Add the nutmeg, cardamom, wine and pepper and simmer for 10 minutes.

3. Add the coconut cream and chick peas (garbanzos) and simmer until the sauce thickens.
4. Serve this dish hot with curries or cold as a salad.

CAN BE FROZEN

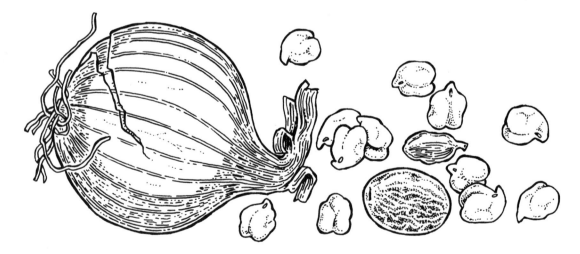

130

Kidney Bean Salad

This dish is vegetarian and high in fibre and low in fat.

Imperial/metric	Serves 4	American
6 oz (170g)	red kidney beans, soaked overnight and drained	1 cup
¼ clove	garlic, crushed/minced	¼ clove
1 tsp	English mustard	1 tsp
1 tbs	wine vinegar	1 tbs
1 tbs	lemon juice	1 tbs
2 tbs	olive oil	2 tbs
	salt	
	freshly ground black pepper	
1	onion, finely chopped	1
1	sweet/green pepper, finely chopped	1
½	small lettuce, washed	½
1 tbs	fresh parsley, finely chopped	1 tbs

1. Put the kidney beans in a pan and cover with water. Bring to the boil and boil rapidly for the first 10 minutes, then cover and simmer for 1-1¼ hours until tender. Drain and put in a bowl to cool.

2. Put the garlic, English mustard, wine vinegar, lemon juice, olive oil, salt and pepper in a clean screw-top jar and shake well to mix.

3. While the beans are still a little warm, toss in the dressing, then leave to cool.

4. Add the onion and pepper to the beans and mix well.

5. Serve the salad on a bed of the lettuce and sprinkle the parsley over the kidney bean salad and chill for 1 hour before serving.

Mixed Bean and Tomato Salad

This dish is low in fat and high in fibre.

Imperial/metric	*Serves 4*	American
8 oz (225g)	mixed dried beans, soaked overnight and drained	2 cups
2	celery sticks/stalks, sliced	2
4	spring onions/scallions, chopped	4
4	medium tomatoes, chopped	4
	For dressing	
¼ pt (140ml)	tomato juice	⅔ cup
1 tbs (15ml)	olive oil	1 tbs
1 tbs (15ml)	lemon juice	1 tbs
1 clove	garlic, crushed/minced	1 clove
2 tbs	chives, chopped	2 tbs
	salt and pepper to taste	

1. Place the beans in a pan and cover with cold water. Add a little salt and simmer for 30-40 minutes until they have softened.

2. Meanwhile, combine all the dressing ingredients in a screw-top jar and shake until thoroughly mixed.

3. When the beans are soft, drain and mix with the dressing while still warm. Leave to cool.

4. Add the celery, spring onions (scallions) and tomatoes and season with salt and pepper to taste.

5. Transfer to a salad bowl and serve.

Winter Salad

This dish is high in fibre and low in fat.

Imperial/metric	Serves 4	American
¼	hard white cabbage	¼
2	carrots, grated	2
2	sticks/stalks celery, chopped	2
2 oz (55g)	sultanas/golden seedless raisins	⅓ cup
2 oz (55g)	English walnuts, chopped	½ cup
1	sweet/red pepper, chopped	1
1 tbs	olive oil	1 tbs
1 tbs	wine vinegar	1 tbs
	pinch dried herbs	
	salt	
	freshly ground black pepper	

1. Grate the cabbage and mix with the carrots, celery, sultanas (golden seedless raisins), walnuts and pepper.

2. Put the remaining ingredients in a screw-top jar and shake well to mix.

3. Toss the salad in the dressing, then serve immediately.

Spring Salad

This dish is high in fibre and low in fat.

Imperial/metric	*Serves 4*	American
1 head	cos/romaine lettuce	1 head
5	spring onions/scallions, sliced	5
	Small bunch radishes, halved	
½	sweet/green pepper, chopped	½
½	sweet/red pepper, chopped	½
2	carrots, grated	2
2 tbs	sunflower seeds	2 tbs
	Dressing	
1 tbs	olive oil	1 tbs
1 tbs	wine vinegar	1 tbs
½ tsp	dried herbs	½ tsp
	or	
1 tsp	fresh herbs, finely chopped	1 tsp
	Freshly ground black pepper	

1. Cut the cos (romaine) lettuce across the leaves into approximately 1-in (2.5-cm) pieces.
2. Put the lettuce in a large bowl with the spring onions (scallions), radishes, peppers, carrot and sunflower seeds.

3. Put the oil, vinegar, herbs and pepper in a clean screw-top jar and shake until well mixed.
4. Toss the salad ingredients in the dressing and chill before serving.

Walnut and Grape Salad

This dish is relatively low in fat.

Imperial/metric	Serves 4	American
1	small iceberg lettuce	1
4 oz (115g)	fresh spinach	3 cups
3 oz (85g)	(English) walnuts	⅔ cup
12 oz (340g)	green grapes, halved and seeded	3 cups
2 tbs (30ml)	vinaigrette dressing (bottled)	2 tbs

1. Separate the lettuce leaves and wash and dry thoroughly.

2. Wash the spinach and dry the leaves well.

3. Tear up the lettuce and spinach leaves by hand.

4. In a large bowl, combine the lettuce and spinach leaves with the walnuts and grapes.

5. Toss the salad gently in the vinaigrette dressing just before serving.

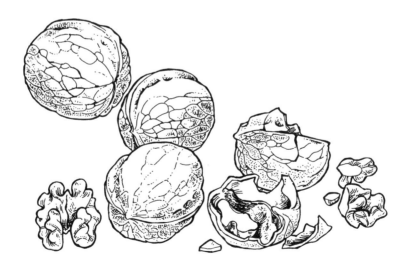

Chapter 12

Desserts

Oaty Apricot Crumble

This dish is high in fibre.

Imperial/metric	*Serves 4*	American
1 lb (455g)	fresh apricots, stoned/pitted and halved	1 lb
4 tbs	water	4 tbs
1 dsp	sugar	2 tsp
2 oz (55g)	sunflower margarine	¼ cup
2 oz (55g)	wholemeal/wholewheat flour	½ cup
1 oz (30g)	rolled oats	¼ cup
1 oz (30g)	demerara sugar	2 tbs

1. Put the apricots, water and sugar in a saucepan and simmer gently until the apricots are soft.

2. Pour the apricots into a lightly greased 2-pt (1.4l/1 quart) casserole dish.

3. Rub the margarine into the flour until it resembles breadcrumbs, then stir in the oats and the sugar.

4. Sprinkle the crumble mixture on top of the apricots and firm down slightly.

5. Bake at 350°F/180°C (Gas Mark 4) for 15-20 minutes.

CAN BE FROZEN
(You can freeze just the cooked apricots or just the crumble mixture or the made up crumble — whatever is most useful.)

Tropical Three Fruit Salad

This dish is high in fibre and low in added sugar.

Imperial/metric	*Serves 4*	American
1	pineapple, whole, fresh, peeled, cored and chopped	1
2	bananas, sliced	2
2	large oranges, peeled and sliced	2
3 tbs	dark rum (optional)	3 tbs

1. Mix the pineapple, bananas and oranges, adding all the juices.

2. Stir in the rum, if used, and chill the salad.

3. Serve with low-fat natural (plain) yoghurt or Greek strained yoghurt.

Luscious Summer Fruit Salad

This dish is high in fibre and low in added sugar.

Imperial/metric	*Serves 4*	American
½ lb (225g)	fresh apricots, halved and stoned/pitted	½ lb
2 tbs	water	2 tbs
2	bananas, sliced	2
2	nectarines, stoned/pitted and sliced	2
2 oz (55g)	seedless green grapes	½ cup
1	orange, peeled and sliced	1
3 tbs	medium sherry	3 tbs

1. Put the apricots and water in a saucepan and poach gently until the fruit is soft but not mushy, then leave to cool.

2. Stir in the banana, nectarine, grapes, orange and sherry.

3. Chill well before serving and serve with low-fat natural (plain) yoghurt or Greek strained yoghurt.

Fruit Kebabs

This dish is high in fibre.

Imperial/metric	*Serves 4*	American
3	bananas	3
8 oz (225g)	pineapple, fresh, cut into chunks	1½ cups
3	peaches	3
3	apples	3
2 tbs	lemon juice	2 tbs
	rind and juice of 1 orange	
2 tbs	clear honey	2 tbs
	pinch mixed spice	

1. Peel the bananas and cut into 1-in (2.5-cm) pieces.
2. Peel and stone (pit) the peaches and cut into chunks.
3. Peel and core the apple and cut into chunks.
4. Place the fruit in a large bowl with the lemon and orange juice. Toss the fruit in the juices to prevent it browning.
5. Thread the fruit onto 4 kebab skewers and brush with the honey.
6. Grill (broil) the kebabs for 6-8 minutes, turning frequently.
7. Dust with the mixed spice and grated orange rind.

Carrot Cake

This cake is high in fibre.

Imperial/metric	*Serves 4*	American
5 oz (140g)	soft brown sugar	¾ cup
7 oz (200g)	self-raising/self-rising wholemeal/wholewheat flour	1¾ cups
2 tsp	baking powder	2 tsp
6 oz (170g)	carrot, grated	1 cup
5 oz (140g)	crushed pineapple	1 cup
2 fl oz (140ml)	sunflower oil	⅔ cup
2	eggs	2

1. Preheat the oven to 350°F/180°C (Gas Mark 4).
2. Put the sugar, flour, baking powder, carrots and pineapple in a large mixing bowl.
3. Mix together the sunflower oil and the eggs and gradually add to the other ingredients, mixing well.

4. Pour the cake batter into a deep 8-in (20-cm) round cake tin (pan) lined with greased greaseproof (waxed) paper and bake for 1 hour until the centre of the cake springs back when lightly pressed. Leave the cake to cool in the tin.

CAN BE FROZEN

Wholemeal (Wholewheat) Scones

This dish is high in fibre and relatively low in fat and added sugar.

Imperial/metric	Makes 8-10 wedges	American
8 oz (225g)	wholemeal/wholewheat self-raising/self-rising flour	2 cups
1½ oz (45g)	margarine	3 tbs
2 oz (55g)	brown sugar	⅓ cup
2-3 tbs	sultanas/golden seedless raisins	2-3 tbs
1	egg, beaten, plus enough semi-skimmed/low-fat milk to make up to ¼ pt (140ml/⅔ cup)	1
1 tsp	sesame seeds	1 tsp

1. Put the flour in a mixing bowl and rub in the margarine until the mixture resembles breadcrumbs.
2. Stir in the sugar and sultanas (golden seedless raisins).
3. Gradually mix in the egg and milk mixture, reserving a little liquid to use as a glaze later. mix well, then knead the mixture lightly on a floured board.

4. Shape into a large, thickish round and put on a greased baking sheet. Brush with the reserved egg and milk and sprinkle the sesame seeds over the top. With a blunt knife, lightly mark out 8-10 wedges.
5. Bake for 15-20 minutes at 425°F/220°C (Gas Mark 7).
6. When baked, place on a cooling rack for a short time, but serve warm.

CAN BE FROZEN
(Re-heat slowly after thawing.)

Useful Addresses

UK

BACUP
121/123 Charterhouse Street, London EC1M
6AA
Tel: 071-608 1661
Outside London for information linkline: 0800
181199
Administration: 071-608 1785

Helps patients, families and friends cope with
and find out more about cancer.

**Breast Care and Mastectomy Association of
Great Britain**
26a Harrison Street, Kings Cross, London
WC1H 8JG
Tel: 071-837 0908

CancerLink
17 Britannia Street, London WC1X 9JN
Tel: 071-833 2451

Cancer Relief Macmillan Fund
Anchor House, 15/19 Britten Street, London
SW3 3TZ
Tel: 071-351 7811

Let's Face It
Christine Piff, 10 Wood End, Crowthorne,
Berkshire RG11 6DQ
Tel: 0344 774405

A contact point for people of any age coping with
facial disfigurement.

Marie Curie Cancer Care
28 Belgrave Square, London SW1X 8QG
Tel: 071-235 3325

The Royal Marsden Hospital
Patient Information Series, Haigh and Hochland
Ltd, International University Booksellers, The
Precinct Centre, Oxford Road, Manchester M13
9QA
Tel: 061-273 4156

Produces a series of booklets for cancer patients
and their relatives on many aspects of cancer.
Topics include chemotherapy, radiotherapy,
cancer of the cervix, breast, ovary, and lung and
problems associated with treatment, such as hair
loss.

The Ulster Cancer Foundation
40-42 Eglantine Avenue, Belfast BT9 6DX
Tel: 0232 663281/2/3
 Helpline: 0232 663439 (09.30-12.30 weekdays)

Irish Cancer Society
5 Northumberland Road, Dublin 4
Tel: 0001 681855, or dial 10 and ask for 'Freefone Cancer' (Ireland only)

Australia

Australian Cancer Society
GPO Box 4708, Sydney, NSW 2001
Tel: 02 211 2599

Breast Cancer Support Services
NSW Cancer Council, GPO Box 7070, Sydney 2001
Tel: 264 8888 (from 11am-2pm)

Cancer Information & Support Society
65 Bay Road, Waverton 2060
Tel: 922 2334

USA

American Cancer Society
Tower Place, 3340 Peachtree Road, NE, Atlanta, GA 30026

Breast Cancer Support Program
1757 Ridge Road, Homewood, IL 60430
Tel: 800 221 2141

Cancer Information Service
Building 31, Room 10A24, 9000 Rockville Pike, Bethesda, MD 20892
Tel: 800 4-CANCER

National Cancer Institute
9000 Rockville Pike, Bethesda, MD 20892

Papanicolaou Cancer Center
PO Box 016960, Miami, FL 33136
Tel: 800 4-CANCER

USC Cancer Center
1721 Griffin Ave, Room 205, Los Angeles, CA 90031
Tel: 800 422 6237

National Cancer Survivors Network
PO Box 4543, Albuquerque, NM 82196
Tel: 505 268 7388

Suggested Reading

General Books on Cancer

Living with Cancer, Jenny Bryan and Joanna Lyall (Penguin Health, 1987)

Understanding Cancer, Which? Books (Consumer's Association and Hodder & Stoughton, 1986)

Cancer: A Guide for Patients and their Families, Chris and Sue Williams (John Wiley & Sons, 1986)

Recipe Books

Low-Fat Cookery, Wendy Godfrey (A Sainsbury Cookbook, J. Sainsbury PLC)

The Low-Fat Gourmet, Caroline Waldegrave (A Sainsbury Cookbook, J. Sainsbury PLC)

The New BBC Diet Book, Dr Barry Lynch (BBC Books)

The Taste of Health: The BBC Guide to Healthy Cooking, Ed. by Jenny Rogers (BBC Books)

Low Fat and No-Fat Cooking, Jackie Applebee (Thorsons)

Nutrition

Healthy Eating, Isabel Skypala (Wisebuy Publications, 1988)

Complementary Diet Books

The Bristol Recipe Book, Sadhaya Rippon, (Century Paperbacks, 1987)

Basic Macrobiotics, Herman Aihara (Japan Publications Inc., 1985)

A Cancer Therapy, Max Gerson (Totality Books Publishers, Del Mar, California, 1977)

Index